Reflections From the Home Team... Go the Distance

Reflections From the Home Team... Go the Distance

David Welter

Xulon Elite

Xulon Press Elite
2301 Lucien Way #415
Maitland, FL 32751
407.339.4217
www.xulonpress.com

EXULON
ELITE

Edited by Xulon Press.

Printed in the United States of America.

ISBN-13: 9781545607572

Dedication

And over all these virtues put on love, which binds them all together in perfect unity. (Colossians 3:14)

This book is written with love for my wife Tricia, my three adult children, John, Rob, and Sarah, their spouses, and my beautiful granddaughters, Grace and Lucy. It hasn't always been easy as you each know, but you have always stood by me, and I couldn't have done it without your unfailing love and support!

Table of Contents

Foreword by Pastor Brian King

The writer and theologian Frederick Buechner has said: "The place God calls you to is the place where your deep gladness and the world's deep hunger meet." My friend, Dave Welter, has found many ways to connect his "deep gladness and the world's deep hunger" while living out his callings as a husband, father, teacher, principal, and coach. It is this latter calling that looms largest in the pages that follow. Dave is the consummate coach and this book provides coaching for people who are facing difficult challenges and who are hungry for hope.

At their best, coaches instruct, encourage, challenge, and develop others in terms of a specific sport or skill set. They help people to envision the future, set goals, persevere through adversity, and succeed. While Dave speaks often of the value of having a "**Home Team**" and frequently uses baseball metaphors to make his points, his insights and encouragement transcend sports and speak to our greatest need as human beings—to be in relationship with God and others. As this book unfolds, you will see this coaching point lifted up time and again as Dave speaks to the inestimable value and support of one's "**Home Team**." As the son of a coach and as a multi-sport athlete in high school and college, I learned early the value of a supportive "**Home Team**" especially when facing difficult obstacles or challenges.

As a sophomore in high school, I participated in two varsity sports at once. On Friday nights I was the fullback for the football team and on Saturdays I would compete as the number four or five man on the Cross Country team. While the results early in the season were largely positive, by the time of the Conference Cross Country Championship, football injuries and inadequate distance conditioning had taken a toll on my running prowess. Having started too fast, I found myself exhausted, defeated, and running in nearly last place on an isolated stretch of the course. Alone, with no other runners, coaches, or fans visible behind me or in front of me, I seriously contemplated quitting — giving up. The pain was just too much, and the challenge of finishing the race ahead and "going the distance" seemed too daunting.

It was in that moment when I was most alone, vulnerable, and overwhelmed that a parent of one of my teammates — a member of my own **"Home Team"** — emerged from a grove of trees shouting words of encouragement and cheering me on. Immediately, I discovered strength I didn't know I had to run faster and farther and finish my race.

In Hebrews 12:1-2, the author writes: "Therefore, since we are surrounded by such a great cloud of witnesses, let us throw off everything that hinders and the sin that so easily entangles. And let us run with perseverance the race marked out for us, fixing our eyes on Jesus."

As I first discovered on that difficult Saturday morning back in 1985 and Dave affirmed early in his cancer fight, we can't meet life's greatest challenges alone. We all need our family, friends, and others to be part of our own "cloud of witnesses" as we "run with perseverance the race marked out for us," or in Dave's words, "find the courage and strength needed to battle through extra innings."

Whatever challenge you may be facing, whatever race you may be running, whatever fight you may be fighting, I pray and trust that Dave's words through this book will emerge at just the right point in your own journey to speak a word of hope and encouragement to you. A word that allows you to discover strength you didn't know you had so that you might "go the distance" toward healing, wholeness, and peace in your own life and circumstances.

Pastor Brian King
Nazareth Evangelical Lutheran Church
Cedar Falls, Iowa

Preface

I am a proud husband and father of three wonderful kids having recently retired from my position as a Jr. High School Principal. Having taught and coached throughout my forty years in education, I am looking forward to my new beginning as a grandfather, baseball scout for the Atlanta Braves, educational consultant, and yes, as a **cancer survivor**.

My life journey has certainly been an adventure, painful at times, but richly rewarding. As a teacher, coach, and school administrator, I have often used God's word as a guiding light when faced with difficult challenges. I've developed a trusting dependence on Him that has been so very helpful for me when questions entered my mind as to why cancer had invaded my body, and how a loving God could allow this to happen to me and my family.

Over the years, I have learned that life is mostly about adjustments. Being a cancer survivor has helped me learn that setting apart some quiet time to be in God's presence is an important adjustment that has become a part of my daily routine. Being near Him has helped me get through some difficult times while strengthening my faith and filling me with peace, particularly during those difficult, often challenging moments.

I have found that processing my cancer journey by writing reflections based on my experiences, and the experiences of those I have come into contact with has been a great comfort for me. Many of the thoughts I share are not original thoughts, but reflect what I have read or discussed with others who may be experiencing similar challenges in their life's journey.

Without question, I have developed a greater compassion for those suffering from this disease and want to reach out to share a message of hope and strength inspiring those who may be facing similar battles. Caring and loving relationships with family, friends, students, and staff throughout my journey have helped provide the courage and the strength I needed to continue fighting the fight. Those precious connections have been so important in my recovery as well as in my daily life moving forward.

I have frequently used baseball analogies and metaphors when writing my reflections since being diagnosed with cancer in 2009. My **"Home Team"** of family, friends, students, and staff have been at my side the whole way. Hence, the title *"Reflections from the Home Team...Go the Distance."* Baseball terminology is, in my opinion, a universal language. It has helped me explain how I have dealt with the ups and downs of treatments. Those adjustments have often been difficult, and despite the challenges, I've done my best to remain positive. Speaking honestly, it hasn't always been easy, just as baseball isn't always easy. The game has taught me much about success and failure, and I have connected the baseball lessons I've learned in my life to my cancer journey as described in the reflections that follow.

A special thanks to all who have been a part of my journey, and to those who have opened their hearts and minds while sharing their thoughts and emotions with me when it is often so hard to do. May these reflections help others find their way when dealing with the struggles each day can bring, while always keeping God's unfailing love at our side.

Introduction

The cancer journey is one that many have experienced either personally or with a family member or loved one. Having the opportunity to share my thoughts and reflections in this book will be for all those who may be experiencing what so often is a raw, emotional experience with cancer. I often asked myself how I might best be able to use my story to provide some hope, comfort, and maybe even a lighter moment or two for those who may be facing a similar battle themselves or with a loved one. As a result of prayerful consideration and encouragement from many on my "**Home Team**," I have decided to transition the thoughts and reflections from my journal into the thoughts and reflections in this book.

I've always done my best to keep things low key and speak from my heart. There certainly have been lots of highs and lows during my cancer journey. However, I'm no longer afraid of what may be ahead because I know God has a plan and will give me what I need to achieve that plan. I'm good with that, whatever it brings, having faith that God has saved me an eternal place on His roster in Heaven.

I have often had a difficult time expressing my thoughts verbally as I tend to get pretty emotional. So, having the opportunity to write and process my thoughts has been important for me. Being an old baseball coach, having my tear ducts leak a little at times hasn't been a bad thing along the way. I see it as just another way to "water the infield" and keep it in good playing condition!

While I progressed in the treatment plan, I made many new connections and reestablished some old ones. As often has been the case in my life, it takes a significant event of some sort to bring me back to the important connections so I am not just depending on myself. All of us experience interruptions in our lives and this was certainly one in mine. I've learned from this experience that some of the most important relationships that I've made came from what I first considered an interruption.

I've also learned that the mission God gives each of us in life is almost always about people and the special connections we make with those who come into our lives. If there is one thing this part of my journey has taught me, it's that difficult times can connect us to others in ways we may never have otherwise realized. Those precious connections not only give us the strength and support needed to survive, but also provide us an opportunity to serve others and their needs.

A letter I received from one of my students shortly after I shared my diagnosis explains just how important those connections can be.

March 3, 2009

Dear Mr. Dave Welter,

Sorry I used your full name, but it's a letter and I figured it would be all right.

When I first moved to Holmes from another school, I thought you were kind of "cheesy," but I sure don't think that now! I was sour when I came to Holmes because I didn't want to leave my old school and friends. Your simple hellos and good mornings meant a lot to me. I can't thank you enough for everything you did to

make me feel better here at school. As I started
making friends here, you still greeted me each
day and talked to me about things we both enjoy
like fishing and hunting. That's cool!

Usually teachers and principals say good
morning for only your first day, but you kept it
up. You have a great optimism and I know you
truly love your students. You made me feel like
I belonged at Holmes, and I have to say, now I
really feel I do belong.

I am a religious person and I want you to
know I will be keeping you in my prayers. I know
you will fight and I know you will survive. My
grandma made it through cancer and she had
only a 20 percent chance of survival. Everyone
thought she wouldn't make it, but I knew she
would! I know after your time for treatments,
you will be back on top again, leading the staff
and students and making others feel welcome
just as you did me.

I'm not very good at this "writing a letter"
thing, so I'm going to sign off for now. Good
luck, Mr. Welter, and thanks for all you did
for me here!

Sincerely, Chris

I'd have to disagree with Chris that he is not good at the
"letter writing thing." His words will always remain embedded
in my heart. As readers process the reflections in my book, I am
hopeful that the thoughts presented will remain in each reader's
heart, just as Chris' words have remained in mine.

Each entry in the book will begin with a transition that will
provide context to the circumstances surrounding each original
reflection. The transition will be followed by an image and

quote which features a central message found in each original reflection. By blending a combination of images and thoughts in my reflections, I have found inspiration and motivation to continue the battle. My hope is that they will provide the same for its readers as well.

Part I

A Life-Changing Event
What's the Plan?

March 2, 2009

I t all began as a typical day. I was planning to celebrate my fifty-fifth birthday with a small gathering of family, but first I had an appointment in Iowa City at University Hospital as a follow up to a bump on my neck that my family doctor discovered during a routine physical. I was referred to Iowa City, and upon arrival, my doctor decided to do a biopsy on the spot.

Within an hour, my life changed. I was diagnosed with stage-three throat cancer and was told this form of cancer has about a 60 percent survival rate. My medical team shared that a treatment plan needed to be determined and implemented quickly to give me the best chance of survival.

My wife, Tricia and I, both went numb. Then my brain kicked into analyzer mode asking:

- *How will this affect my family and my job?*
- *How do I tell others?*
- *What's the plan for treatment?*

These were generally all things that I would take on and try to solve on my own. I was feeling overwhelmed and needed to find a way to deal with it all. It was at that point that the numbness turned into raw emotion and the tears began to flow. I have to admit—those tears flow regularly even yet.

We arrived back home, and I took care of some work related responsibilities that evening. First, I reported to supervise our annual Spring Show at school, while all the time thinking this may be my last. As my mind drifted throughout the following weekend, I recalled that my doctors had given me some direction on what my schedule would look like over the next six months. So, I turned to what I have always been comfortable doing when faced with difficult situations.

I began journaling my thoughts.

I began thinking and deciding how to share my *reflections* with family, friends, my students, and staff. What follows now in this book are those journal reflections with some spiritual insight, encouraging quotes from wise and thoughtful famous and unknown people, and some suggestions on action and attitudinal steps you might consider taking to help you or a friend walk through this life-changing event—cancer. I invite you to consider journaling your walk for yourself and perhaps to share later with others as I have done. It's very helpful and healing to keep a journal.

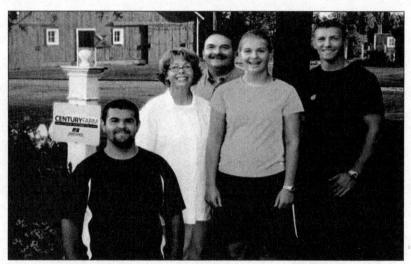

The Core Strength of My Journey—My Family]

Reflection 1

Sharing the News

"It is with a heavy heart I share this message...."

March 2, 2009

As has happened many times over my ten years in this building, the staff and students at our school have always pulled together when troubled times faced them. Often, our human desires of "wanting to know" and "wanting to share" can interfere with an individual's right to privacy. I have always respected an individual's right to privacy, and have allowed each person the opportunity to share as much or as little as they choose to share. Each situation is always unique, and a good place to start so that misinformation does not begin circulating is with the facts. Given that attitude, I choose to share the following information with my school staff and students.

> *"It is with a heavy heart I share this message. I returned late last Tuesday from Iowa City with my wife Tricia. Following several weeks of testing, I have been diagnosed with a form of small cell throat cancer. The doctors feel I am currently in stage-three, and have shared that this form of cancer has a sixty percent survival*

rate. We will determine the extent of that with further testing this week. I am now working with a Medical Team in Iowa City to prepare a course of treatment which will last seven to eight weeks and will report there to begin testing for my regimen of treatment on Tuesday, March 3.

I will have to remain in Iowa City throughout the treatment period with the possibility of coming home on weekends if I am up to it. The recovery period may take an additional eight weeks if things go well. My prayers are that they will. I am a survivor, and I have a loving family, friends, student body and staff for support. I also have faith that God has a plan for me, and I am placing myself in His hands.

Being a baseball guy, that sixty percent survival rate would translate into a .600 batting average, so I'll take those odds and begin the fight! As I leave to begin the battle, I'd ask a favor from each of you. I'd ask that you pull together as you always have to work with each other to make this year finish out in a positive way. In my absence, please give those stepping in to help manage the building in my absence your utmost respect and cooperation. I promise you that I will fight to achieve a victory over this disease so that I can continue to fulfill my life's goal of seeing each and every one of you become successful in life.

Always remember, I love each of you and will always do what I can to help you become the best person you can be. My hope is that we can make today a good, productive day. My wish is that we all take one day at a time, making the most of our individual talents and gifts knowing that when we lay our heads on our pillows at night, we will rest well because we have used up all our potential for that day making a positive difference.

-Mr. Welter

March 5, 2009

My doctors had given me some direction on what my schedule might look like over the next six months, so I turned my thoughts to how I would manage a new game plan that would now become a part of my life. I knew that plan needed to include a physical, emotional, and spiritual component in order to be successful. I had developed such a plan when I became a principal in 1989, and those components just needed some dusting off.

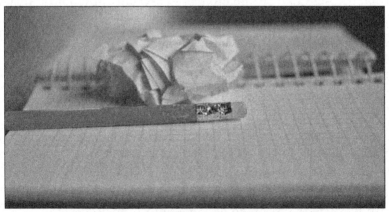

"My game plan is to seek each day as an opportunity to begin with a clean slate."

As often has been the case in my life, it generally takes a significant event of some sort to bring me back to the important connections and goals I had established. I was tempted to

isolate myself totally from everything in order to focus only on those components when I realized that I desperately needed the support of others to make the physical, emotional, and spiritual factors work in my plan. I needed my family, friends, students, and staff to hold me accountable, while providing me the strength I needed to, *"Go the Distance!"*
March 5, 2009

I have been back and forth between Cedar Falls and Iowa City the past few days. The plan at this point is to go in for Oral Surgery Thursday morning at University Hospitals in Iowa City. I have an 8:00 a.m. appointment. So, I am on the road again!

I must have my four wisdom teeth pulled prior to treatment. This is a standard procedure with head, neck, and throat cancer. Guess I learn something new every day. I've worked hard to keep my teeth in good shape, but I have to do what I have to do.

It will take seven to ten days to heal before we can begin practice sessions of radiation and chemotherapy. Those treatments will then start immediately after, probably around spring break. I need to share that my emotional bank was running a deficit Monday morning when I came to school.

It has been a rough few weeks for my family and me. I also need to say that by the end of the day, my emotional bank was overflowing because of the support and prayers you all have been offering for my family and me! I can't tell you how much that means as I train for this fight. I am preparing physically, emotionally, and spiritually for the battle. I know that on some days, one or more of those ingredients may drop off a bit. If so, I'll work on the others to pick me up!

My love for all of you runs deep, and I know that all of you are willing to help as needed. That is greatly appreciated. I do want you to know that the coach in me has surfaced again, imagine that! I have polished off the "game plan" that I developed when I first became a Principal a few years back. I want to share it with you so you can continue to hold me accountable as I move forward.

> *My game plan is to seek each day as an opportunity to begin with a clean slate. I will avoid neither risk nor responsibility nor fear failure, and I will spend each day using up all my potential.*

> *I will seek to build complementary relationships with family, friends, and associates. I will make daily deposits in the emotional bank accounts of others and in some way, find a way to say thanks to God every day.*

> *I prefer to let my work speak for me and believe in achieving visibility through my productivity.*

> *I will always deal with others with honesty and integrity, tolerance, compassion, evenness, and consideration.*

> *I will dedicate my remaining years to helping others find purpose in their lives, ensuring that my influence on others is consistent with my values and principles.*

> *I will accomplish this "game plan" keeping a daily balance with my spiritual, family, physical, social-emotional, and job responsibilities.*

If I drop off on some of my game plan, please be ready to remind me of it! This community is one I am so proud to call home!

An Encouraging Attitude

"My game plan is to seek each day as an opportunity to begin
with a clean slate.
I will avoid neither risk nor responsibility nor fear failure,
and I will spend each day using up all my potential."
–Dave Welter

A Spiritual Insight

"I have fought the good fight,
I have finished the race,
I have kept the faith."
(Paul writing about his life's journey in 2 Timothy 4:7)

A Step to Consider

Gather a support team around you and make a plan.

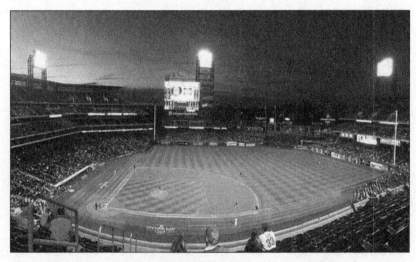

"I will be using baseball terminology to keep you posted".

Reflection 2

The Home Team vs. the Visiting Team

March 13, 2009

C oaching and educating young people has formed the core of my life over the past forty years. Considering the passion and love I have felt for my students and staff during that time, I decided I wanted to use my situation as a teaching opportunity to model a positive mindset for anyone who may be facing not only cancer, but any number of challenging situations in their lives.

Given my passion for coaching and my love of baseball, I have decided to communicate my thoughts and emotions using baseball and sports to help speak to others in a creative, metaphorical way. The use of baseball analogies provides a common thread and theme throughout my reflections. Using baseball terminology has also allowed me to stay in my comfort zone while drawing parallels that provide encouragement for readers who may find themselves or a loved one in a struggle similar to mine. As people often need inspiration in finding any bit of hope they may see in others in a similar situation, my desire is to provide examples of that through the use of baseball analogies and metaphors in the following reflections.

I have had a number of requests to update my progress from family, friends, students, athletes, staff, and parents. After a lot of thought and given my respect for personal privacy, I have decided to keep you updated on my progress as I deem appropriate be using baseball terminology.

In my opinion, baseball terminology is a universal language. It also helps me explain how I will relate the ups and downs of the treatments that lie ahead. From this point on, **Welter** will be designated the **Home Team**, and *Cancer* will be designated the **Visiting Team**.

The Start of the Game

It began as I reported to my routine Spring Training physical in February, 2009. I was getting my routine checkup so I could be cleared to report with pitchers and catchers as I do every spring to prepare for the upcoming season. My Home Team doctor and I discussed an unusual bump on the left side of my neck and he thought it best to refer me to a specialist. The specialist made a diagnosis and thought the bump could be surgically removed with just a few potential complications. He referred me to University of Iowa Hospital for the surgery because of their expertise in head, neck, and throat issues. As the specialists reviewed previous testing, they noticed some additional concerns on the MRI and ordered additional testing.

I felt like if I drank a glass of water, I could be used as a sprinkler system for the infield given the number of needles that had been injected in me. As the results were analyzed, my **Home Team** surgeon determined I was suffering from a form of small cell throat cancer, and that I had already progressed to stage three. She immediately assembled a team of doctors to help plan a course of treatment, which I have been preparing for over the past two weeks.

I will pursue both radiation and chemotherapy treatments for the next eight weeks, and if that does not eliminate the **Visiting Team** from my body, we will then turn to surgery. I have the advance scouting report from my **Home Team** doctors, and it indicates that the **Visiting Team** has an arsenal of nasty pitches and heavy hitting symptoms not only from the disease itself, but also from the treatments. The first step includes having any teeth surgically removed that could present a problem down the road, even though all my teeth are currently healthy. I had eight teeth removed last Thursday (four wisdom teeth and four molars). This was done with no sedation as I was fighting a bad cold and couldn't be put under. I am currently healing before I can proceed with radiation treatments. Healing will not occur during radiation. I have several appointments scheduled in Iowa City on Friday to determine if I am sufficiently healed and virus free so I can move forward.

As the **Visiting Team** snuck into town around my fifty-fifth birthday, little did it realize the amount of support the **Home Team** had as the upcoming contest was announced. The outpouring of support and love from family, friends, students, athletes, and parents has been overwhelming. As one of my heroes, Lou Gehrig once said when he was faced with a similar battle: "Today, I feel like the luckiest man on the face of the earth." I truly feel that because of the love and support all of you have generated for my family and me.

The **Home Team** has a definite home field advantage as we move into the next phase of the contest. The **Visiting Team** loaded the bases in the top of the first, but my **Home Team** shut them out with a great game plan, while scoring one run in the bottom half of the first inning! The score at the end of one full inning of play is: **Home Team 1, Visitor 0!**

Remember, take each day one at a time and be as productive as you can be! I love each of you and I continue to appreciate your thoughts and prayers.

An Encouraging Attitude

15

"Take each day one at a time and be as productive as
you can be!"
–Dave Welter

A Spiritual Insight

"Therefore do not worry about tomorrow,
for tomorrow will worry about itself.
Each day has enough trouble of its own."
(Jesus teaching in Matthew 6:34)

A Step to Consider

Don't let the **Visiting Team** dictate your emotions.
Be positive and proactive, not negative and reactive in your
strategy to fight cancer.
No matter what thoughts come your way, you can overcome
them to accomplish your task. Thoughts will come and go,
just stay in the game and keep moving forward.

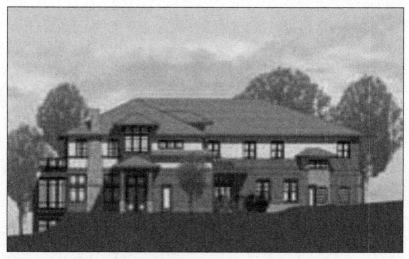
"Hope Lodge; a blessing for my family and me."]

Reflection 3

Be Joyful in Hope

March 20, 2009

One of the many concerns I had when discussing treatments with my **Home Team** doctors was how to manage travel and accommodations throughout my eight weeks of treatments. Given that treatments were scheduled every day, Monday through Friday in Iowa City, the travel became a major concern. It was an hour and forty-minute drive from Cedar Falls to Iowa City. My team of doctors helped me resolve that issue by arranging my stay at Hope Lodge in Iowa City. That way, my wife Tricia could stay at home and be with our family during the week as I received treatments. If I felt up to it, I was allowed to come home on weekends to be with family. What a blessing for both my family and me!

I have now been cleared to begin treatments. I had a trial run with radiation on Friday, March 20, and everything appears to be ready to go. A special mask has been developed to cover my head and neck area when receiving the radiation. That mask allows my head and neck to be secured so that no movement takes place during the radiation treatments. I will report Sunday, March 22, to check into the Hope Lodge in Iowa City where I will begin the second inning of this contest. Hope Lodge is a service funded by the American Cancer Society and is a wonderful place where cancer treatment patients can interact and receive support during their treatment. I feel fortunate to have such an opportunity!

Monday morning begins with a three-hour chemotherapy session followed by radiation. I had to share with my family that if I turned green and got more muscular when agitated, beware because the "Hulk" has nothing on me! This may provide me with more than just warning track power!

An Encouraging Attitude

Special thanks to Mrs. Talbot and all her students who shared their Teeth Tales with me!
It has helped take a "bite" out of my treatments! Love each and every one of you!
- Dave Welter

A Spiritual Insight

"Be joyful in hope,
patient in affliction,
faithful in prayer."
(Paul's instructions for dealing with life's difficulties
Romans 12:12)

A Step to Consider

Remember to take each day one at a time, making it productive.
The nature of hope is that it refers to something in the future, something "not yet."
If patience is not a strong point, we can ask the Holy Spirit to help us wait in His presence.
While we wait for what we may be hoping for, we can rejoice in God's loving company.

Part II

The Grind
Keep Your Positive Focus!

March 27, 2009

With the daily regimen of treatments came a number of physical, emotional, and spiritual challenges. I began reading as much as I could get my hands on to help deal with the situation I found myself in. Relating to others who had faced or were facing similar journeys became a priority. Meeting a number of people in the treatment center taught me that this disease does not discriminate. The fear having cancer can generate makes you dig deep into your soul to figure out what your true priorities are.

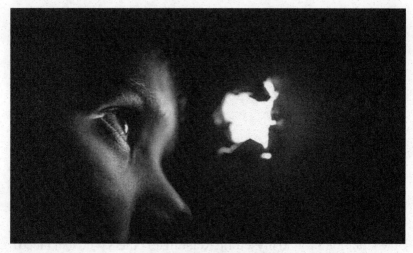

Focus Rather Than Fear!

"To be afraid offers a priceless education, and it makes you know more about yourself and your priorities than most people. Keep your priorities in order and continue to ask more of yourself each day as a person as you take one day at a time. Never give up!"
- Lance Armstrong from his book, *It's Not About the Bike, My Journey Back to Life*

Reflection 4

Annoying the Visiting Team

March 27, 2009

The second inning began Monday morning, March 23, with the **Visiting Team** coming to bat carrying a power packed line-up. Monday started with a three-hour chemo session that extended into six hours, as they had to slow down my assimilation of the drugs. The chemotherapy treatment contained some pretty potent stuff, including platinum. Might be used for a Gold Glove award later in the contest. If my 401 K goes bust, I can harvest myself out for retirement!

I did okay Monday, but had some real nausea issues Tuesday and Wednesday. Again, the **Visiting Team** loaded the bases, and the "chemo demons" were out to get me Tuesday night, but failed to score as the **Home Team** training staff provided some prescriptions to keep the visitors from crossing home plate! I've been receiving radiation every day, and it seems to be annoying the **Visitors'** "dugout" in my throat. My taste buds are toast and I'm getting a terrible sore throat. Anyway, I'm getting through this knowing that if the **Home Team** is feeling this way, the **Visitors** are getting the worst end of it because they are on the road! Keeps me going! Miss you guys! Hold the fort down until I can return healthy, wealthy (with my platinum), and wiser.

I've been doing a lot of reading. Lance Armstrong makes some great observations about his fight with cancer that sure are hitting home with me in his book, *It's Not About the Bike, My Journey Back to Life.* I have met a lot of people here this week suffering far greater than I am, and I agree with him that this disease does not discriminate or listen to the odds. It can decimate a strong person with a wonderful attitude, while it somehow miraculously spares a weaker person who is resigned to failure.

As I sit in my treatments, I have observed it is not about worthiness, as I am no more or less valuable than the person sitting next to me in the chemo center. It is, as Armstrong says, the fact that you are staring into a mystery about your future that makes this significant no matter who we are.

The score at the end of two full innings of play is: **Home Team - 2, Visitors - 0!**

An Encouraging Attitude

"I'm not sure just yet how my story will end,
but I will guarantee you that nowhere in it will it ever read
I gave up!"
-Dave Welter

A Spiritual Insight

"[The Lord] gives strength to the weary
and increases the power of the weak."
(The Prophet offering comfort and encouragement to God's
people in Isaiah 40:29)

A Step to Consider

Reading has brought me much encouragement and comfort
on my journey.
As E.B. White shares: "A library is a good place to go
when you feel unhappy,
for there, in a book, you may find encouragement and comfort.
A library is a good place to go when you feel
bewildered or undecided,
for there, in a book, you may have your question answered.
Books are good company, in sad times and happy times,
for books are people –
people who have managed to stay alive by hiding
between the covers of a book."
Read an encouraging book and be inspired by a survivor!

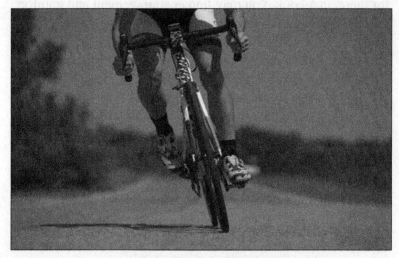
Training for the Comeback

"I am also training… not for the Tour de France, but to return to the Tour de Holmes faster than anyone else!"
- *Dave Welter paraphrasing* Lance Armstrong from his book, *It's Not About the Bike, My Journey Back to Life*

Reflection 5

Stick to the Game Plan

March 31, 2009

The third inning began with some good news and some challenging news. I met with my team of doctors on Monday, March 31, following some lab work that had been done. The good news is that my neck and throat tumors are softening and beginning to get smaller after only one week of treatments. That was uplifting news! I then went in for my weekly chemo treatment and had a very bad reaction to the Taxol and its delivery agent. It took around 60 minutes to get that under control and the doctors once again slowed the delivery making it an 8-hour session of chemo. I hung tough, though, and it reinforced my philosophy over the years of respecting your opponent and staying focused when you get a lead in a game. I also reminded myself to stick to the game plan!

My training team has developed a good game plan and it seems to be creating some dissention in the **Visitor's** dugout. They seem to be wanting to escape the dugout at all hours of the day and night. I've had some intense coughing going on while attempting to clear my throat. I also had a meeting Thursday with my team of doctors and did some baseline testing of swallowing. Then I met with a speech pathologist who discussed a possible food peg in the next week or so. All part of the plan to defeat the **Visiting Team**!

As I continue to read, I came across another interesting point made by Lance Armstrong in his book, *It's Not About the Bike, My Journey Back to Life*. In his comeback training regimen following cancer, Lance made the following statement that I think applies in all our lives with regard to education and it's relevance in our daily lives. Many times I get asked at school, "So, when am I ever going to use any of this stuff?" Here is Lance's quote:

> *"I geeked out. I tackled the problem of the Tour de France as if I were in math class, science class, chemistry class and nutrition class all rolled into one. I did computer calculations that balanced my body weight and my equipment weight with the potential velocity of the bike in various stages, trying to find the equation that would get me to the finish line faster than anyone else. I kept careful computer graphs of my training rides, calibrating the distances, wattages and thresholds."*
>
> *"Even eating became mathematical. I measured my food intake. I kept a small scale in the kitchen and weighed the portions of pasta and bread. Then I calculated my wattages versus my caloric intake so I knew precisely how much to eat each day, how many calories to burn, so that the amount coming in would be less than my output, and I would lose weight."*

Now for me, that is relevant learning! I am also training, not for the Tour de France, but to return to the "Tour de Holmes" faster than anyone else! I am using many of the same equations

with my doctors as I plan my daily diet to keep weight on, and keep up my strength throughout all nine innings.
The score at the end of three full innings of play: **Home Team - 3, Visitors - 0.**

An Encouraging Attitude

I worked with my training team to develop a good game plan
to create some dissention in the **Visitor's** dugout.
- Dave Welter

A Spiritual Insight

"If any of you lacks wisdom [to guide him
through a decision or circumstance],
he is to ask of [our benevolent] God,
who gives to everyone generously
and without rebuke *or* blame, and it will be given to him."
(Wisdom from James, the brother of Jesus in James 1:5[1])

A Step to Consider

Use education and its relevance in our daily lives to
think outside the box
and tackle problems by using **all** the resources
at your disposal.

---

[1] Amplified Bible Translation

29

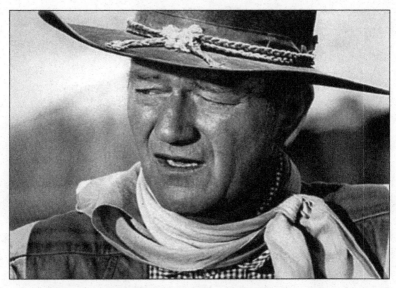

"Courage is being scared to death-but saddling up anyway." - John Wayne.

Reflection 6

Mental Toughness

April 9, 2009

This segment of my treatments was definitely filled with highs and lows. My initial results showed some progress in shrinking the tumors in my throat, but the treatments that were making that possible were sending the rest of my system into chaos! I hung my cap on the fact that if I was feeling this bad, the cancer cells in my throat had to be feeling much worse. It seemed the coughing fits I was having at night was an attempt by the **Visitors** to get out of town under the cover of darkness!

The chemo "demons" were beginning to appear at night, causing some pretty intense nausea and the radiation was really impacting my swallowing and voice. I began to develop a great relationship with my radiation nurse who helped me find ways to deal with some of the side effects of treatment. I readily welcomed her as an important part of my **Home Team**! She was compassionate, yet firm in her expectations while guiding me between treatments. I told her she would make a great coach. She offered a smile, sharing she preferred being a nurse because generally, nurses have no parents to deal with!

Lance Armstrong's book and a good friend who visited me during the week provided me with additional inspiration and a good dose of mental toughness, which was just what I needed at this stage of my treatments.

The fourth inning began with my weekly lab work and visitation with the **Home Team** trainers and doctors. I was experiencing some ulcers in my throat and mouth from the radiation that presented some problems with eating and talking, so the doctors prescribed some medication to help with that. I guess I needed to trim down for the season, and there may be some who would be alright if I were fairly quiet over the next six weeks, so I'll take it all in stride!

The good news is my labs indicate the tumors continue to diminish in size from treatments. My oncologist shared today, "I hate to have to put you through this, but you will be rewarded in the end."

I quoted him 1 Corinthians 9:24: "Do you not know that in a race all the runners run, but only one gets the prize? Run in such a way as to get the prize." I shared that we both want that prize at the end of the game and I am running to win this race!

It's still hard getting any consistent sleep due to the throat issues and congestion. Might take a hose to the dugout and clean it out one day soon. My radiation nurse, Peggy, has adopted me as her surrogate son during my treatments and I affectionately refer to her as mom. She suggested I rinse and gargle with meat tenderizer to help with the pain and healing in my mouth and throat. She shared this was a strategy they have recently come across to assist patients with neck and throat cancer. Being an educator, I asked if that was research based or Heloise based and like a true mom she said a little of both, **so try it!** Since it feels like my mouth and throat have been grilled, I guess it makes sense to try.

As I finished the Armstrong book, I wanted to share a reflection that I have in common with Lance as we both have faced a similar situation. People have often asked him about his quote, "Given a choice between cancer and winning the Tour de France, I'd choose the cancer." He explains that he wouldn't have learned all he did if he hadn't had to contend with the cancer and couldn't have won even one Tour without what it taught him.

For example, he trained hard before his illness, he was never lazy, but after the cancer, he did even more. Lance shared it even taught him how to cope with losing, whether health, a home, or an old sense of self. Cancer forced both of us to develop a plan for living, and that in turn taught us both how to develop smaller goals to achieve those plans. Take my advice, don't wait for a major life event to happen to you, make a plan for your life and set it out in small attainable goals. Take each day one at a time, and do your best to make it productive!

By the way, I did take the time to watch my Atlanta Braves defeat the World Champion Philadelphia Phillies on opening day! Go Braves!

John Wayne, one of my favorite classic actors also had a battle with cancer. Ironically, a good friend delivered one of his famous quotes to me on a wall hanging here at Hope Lodge on Tuesday, right after I had just finished a combined 9-hour chemo and radiation session.

"Courage is being scared to death-but saddling up anyway." - John Wayne

I have it posted on my wall as a reminder of the drive and focus needed for each day!

An Encouraging Attitude

"I want that prize at the end of the game, so I am running to win this race!"
- Dave Welter

A Spiritual Insight

"Do you not know that in a race all the runners run, but only one gets the prize?
Run in such a way as to get the prize."
(Paul's advice in 1 Corinthians 9:24)

A Step to Consider

Don't wait for a major life event to happen to you, make a plan for your life and set it out in small attainable goals—
starting today.

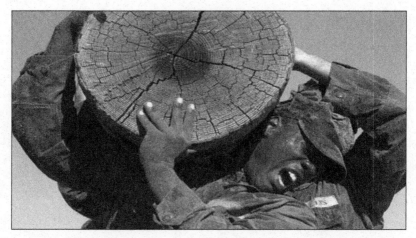

Some "Never Think Quit" Training Strategies

Reflection 7

One Pitch, One Inning at a Time

April 17, 2009

I started off the fifth inning with my 7:00 a.m. lab draws at the Cancer Center. My radiation doctor, my oncologist and my surrogate mother, nurse Peggy met to discuss my progress. My neck and throat tumors continue to diminish in size and were flattening and softening which is all very positive. I asked the doctors where I stood with regard to reaching my goal of being cancer free and they shared that we will not be able to determine that until roughly three months after treatment when they run my next PET scan to determine if I still have cancer cells in my body. Then, there will be approximately a five-year window to see if it returns in a similar or different form.

Just as in baseball, I have to be patient and take it one pitch and one inning at a time with each day providing a fresh and positive opportunity to get the most out of that day. I now realized I would be in this game for the long haul, so I needed some additional inspiration to adjust my plans for the long-term. That inspiration arrived when my oldest son John brought me the book *Lone Survivor* written by Navy Seal Marcus Luttrell. It was one of the most remarkable stories of survival I have ever read and provided me just the right mindset I required at this stage of my journey.

Marcus Luttrell asked his instructor, a man who was respectfully referred to by his first name, "Reno" about some of the harsh training strategies employed by the Navy Seals. Reno's reply has stuck with me.

> *"Marcus, the body can take damn near anything. It's the mind that needs training. Can you cope with unfairness and setback and come back with your jaw set, still determined, and swearing to God you will never quit? That's what we are looking for."* **- Reno**

I was determined to battle through the issues that the radiation treatments were causing me. Holding off inserting a food PEG in order to swallow was one of those challenges. The advantage of a food PEG is that you can maintain the nourishment and hydration needed to sustain yourself during treatments. The disadvantage is that by using the food PEG, you lose the capabilities of swallowing along with the use of your neck, throat, and tongue muscles. Not a good option!

I decided to take the "Navy Seal" approach Marcus described so often in his book. I chose to fight through the neck and throat pain by eating and drinking religiously without the PEG. We all agreed to allow that to happen unless I continued to lose more weight and risk dehydration. However, the doctors warned me that only five percent of their patients make it without a Food PEG.

My father is a Marine Corps Veteran, having served in the Korean War while surviving the Chosen Few Reservoir experience there. My oldest son John is currently a Federal Agent with the elite BORSTAR Unit of the US Border Patrol. Both have been through similar training and experiences, so it helps motivate me to battle my issues with the same mental toughness each of them have displayed.

Instructor Reno also provided some relevant information for me with regard to caring for my body during these times and how it parallels the rigorous training the Seals had to endure.

"The mantra was simple-you take care of your body like the rest of your gear. Keep it well fed and watered, between one and two gallons a day. Start no discipline without a full canteen. That way, your body will take care of you when you begin to ask serious questions of it. Because there is no doubt that in the coming months, you will be asking serious questions of it!" - **Reno**

I plan to take Instructor Reno's advice, staying mentally tough and determined, while never quitting and keeping my canteen full before the start of each inning in this game!

The score after five complete innings of play: **Home Team - 5, Visitors - 0.**

An Encouraging Attitude

"I have to be patient and take it one pitch and
one inning at a time
with each day providing a fresh and positive opportunity
to get the most out of that day." -Dave

A Spiritual Insight

"Therefore we do not become discouraged [spiritless,
disappointed, or afraid].
Though our outer self is [progressively] wasting away,
yet our inner *self* is being [progressively] renewed
day by day."[2]

---

[2] Taken from the Amplified Translation of the Bible

(Paul's call to endure in spite of attacks against our bodies
and minds in 2 Corinthians 4:16)

A Step to Consider

Our walk on this earth is often plodding and heavy.
We need to take it one step at a time clinging to His hand for
strength and direction.
Take care of your body like the rest of your gear.
Keep it well fed and watered.
Start no discipline without a full canteen.

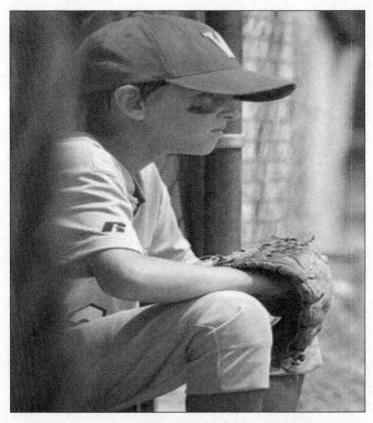

"Mr., when are they going to let you go back outside to play?

Reflection 8

A Little Guy Named Taylor

April 24, 2009

This week began as a typical week filled with blood draws and testing. I began to notice a number of new faces checking in on my progress each day. It seemed my **Home Team** of doctors wanted a number of interns to come in and observe me. I took the opportunity to share a smile or two with them. I finally asked why I was getting so much attention and being asked so many questions.

One of the interns replied, "We generally don't see patients this far along in treatments without food pegs and pain meds. We are wondering what you are doing differently than the others."

I shared with them that I was doing nothing more than what I'm told to do...RELIGIOUSLY! I also shared Marcus Luttrel's quote that "the body can take damn near anything; it's the mind we have to train!" I asked the doctors that if I was to be a case study, maybe we could name it, *"How to stay chilled while being grilled using meat tenderizer!"* They didn't think it would get published, though.

My labs show that my resistance is next to nothing at this time, which is normal given the chemo and radiation. I also had another bad reaction to the chemo on Monday, but seemed to get through the side effects by week's end. Swallowing and talking are still an issue, and I'm down about forty pounds, so I have to monitor calories and hydration carefully. All part of the game plan to win this contest!

Speaking of winning this contest, my oncologist feels good about the shrinking of the tumors in my neck. He feels I am making good progress and getting better! (Even though he says I may not feel like it right now). That put a lift in my spirits!

Another thing really gave me a lift was on Tuesday, when I was at the hospital pharmacy picking up a prescription. A little guy named Taylor, I'd say about third grade, was waiting with his mom. He too had cancer, fighting leukemia, I learned when we talked. He was playing with a rubber baseball, which of course caught my attention.

We began to visit and naturally began a game of catch with each other while waiting. I had to demonstrate some of the famous ball tricks I used back in my playing days. He was quite amused by that.

We were having fun when he point blank asked me, "Mr., when are they going to let you go back outside to play?"

I thought about it, then shared I had about three weeks of treatments left and some recovery time after that, but then I would get to go back out and play.

"How about you?" I asked him looking at his mom. "About the same," she answered. So, we finished our game of catch and wished each other good luck on our journeys. I really hoped this young man got a chance to go back out and play!

That conversation put it in perspective for me, too. I'm ready to win this thing so I can get back outside and play! Thanks Taylor for giving me just the emotional lift I needed! I'd also like to send a special thanks to Mr. Carter and his Health class for all the notes and cards. They really helped lift my spirits this week!

The score after six complete innings of play is now: **Home Team - 6, Visitors - 0!**

An Encouraging Attitude

"I'm ready to win this thing so I can get back outside
and play!"
- **Dave Welter**

A Spiritual Insight

"In everything set them an example by doing what is good."
(Instructions from Paul in Titus 2:7)

A Step to Consider

*"How to stay chilled while being grilled using
meat tenderizer!"* – Dave Welter
Keep your sense of humor!

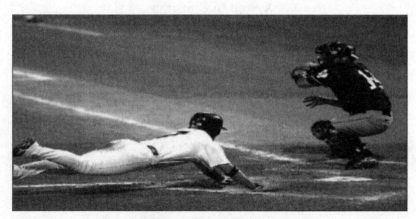

I Plan to Go the Distance

Reflection 9

Be Sure the Last Man Is Out!

May 1, 2009

The seventh inning started off as always with my lab work at the University of Iowa Cancer Center. I had a good conference with my doctors Monday morning where I received the news that today was my last chemo day! The plan was to cut chemo treatments by one given the progress I have made with the shrinking of my tumors. I still have seven radiation treatments left, though.

I had a camera tour of my neck and throat with my radiation doctor. It was like a clip from *Journey to the Center of the Body*. I watched it on a big screen as she was snapping photos inside my throat and neck. She is very pleased with my progress, noting my tonsils, voice box, and tongue are now distinguishable, (without tumors). It appears that only dead tissue and scar tissue remain where the tumors were located. That was very encouraging!

However, the radiation and chemo that are designed to kill off any new baby cells that may mutate from the original cancer, also kill off my white cells, which help with resistance. I just have to be careful not to get infected since something as simple as a common cold could put me in critical condition.

The news was all good, but I am completely drained physically and emotionally. My energy level and emotional bank are running nearly on empty. However, I have a very special weekend with family to look forward to that definitely helped restore my mindset and fighting spirit to its proper place. Many of the loving connections that I had maintained throughout treatments seemed to all come together for me at just the right time.

The weekend schedule includes an engagement party for my son John and his fiancé Shannon, my daughter Sarah's confirmation, and receiving a handmade quilt from my students and staff. The love and energy generated by these people and events help me realize my **Home Team** and I had the **Visiting Team** on the run! Who needs energy drinks when you are surrounded by that kind of love!

The weekend at home went very well. I'm tired, but in a very good way! I had another bad reaction to the chemo on Monday. I'm glad to be done with that part of the treatment process. Swallowing and talking still are an issue along with radiation burns to my neck and throat area, and I'm down about forty-five pounds. I have to continue to monitor calories and hydration carefully. All part of the game plan to win this contest!

Special thanks to all of you Holmes student-staff quilters for my personalized quilt. Reading the names and comments on each of your blocks has lifted my spirits immensely! Even though I am physically drained, my spirits remain high because of the continued prayers, warm thoughts, and kind-hearted acts directed toward my family and me. We all express our thanks and love to you for that!

I have one week of treatments left before earning a break to begin my recuperation from the drain it has taken on me. That will run four to six weeks depending on how my body recovers and the lab results that come back. I am ever optimistic that things will work out according to God's plan for me.

The hardest part of that time will be staying away from people to avoid possible infections, but I'll get through that as well.

I have been continuing my reading and found a quote in *Shoeless Joe*, the novel by W.P. Kinsella that inspired the movie, *Field of Dreams*. That quote sums up my feeling about baseball and life.

> "Baseball is the most perfect of games, solid, true, pure and precious as diamonds. If only life were so simple. Within the baselines anything can happen. Tides can reverse; oceans can open. That's why they say; the game is never over until the last man is out. Colors can change, lives can alter, and anything is possible in this gentle, flawless, loving game." — W.P. Kinsella (Shoeless Joe)

The score after seven complete innings of play: **Home Team - 7, Visitors – 0!**

An Encouraging Attitude

I plan to **go the distance** in this game as both life and baseball are as precious as diamonds.
I want to be sure the last man on the **Visiting Team is out!**

A Spiritual Insight

"For I know the plans I have for you," declares the LORD,
"plans to prosper you and not to harm you,
plans to give you hope and a future."
(Jeremiah 29:11)

A Step to Consider

Pray that today when something doesn't go your way,
you will regroup quickly, let it go, and move onward.
Remain ever optimistic that things will work out
according to God's plan.

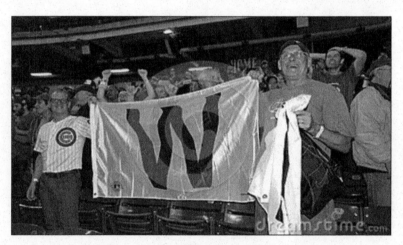

"I couldn't have done it without all of you!"

Reflection 10

Nearing Home

May 8, 2009

As I entered the final innings of my contest in Iowa City, I felt both tremendous highs and incredible lows. The feeling that I was winning the fight was exhilarating, yet my body told me it had endured just about enough. My nurses kept cheering me on, and we had a laugh or two along the way, which really helped. They were always true professionals and knew how to help me cope both physically and emotionally.

> *"From an emotional standpoint, I couldn't have done it without all of you! That includes family, friends, students, and staff. My family and I are most appreciative of the comforting words, kind acts, and daily prayers offered for us throughout this process."* – Dave Welter

The eighth inning started off as always with my lab work at the University of Iowa Cancer Center. I had a good conference with my doctors where I received the news I would be finishing my radiation treatments on Friday, May 8. My radiation doctor feels very good about my progress so far, and I do as well despite the fact I am physically exhausted and worn down.

The side effects of chemo and radiation are pretty dramatic, and I know it will take some time to recover. I have continued to do my best to workout daily despite feeling pretty exhausted and the doctors feel that will be a plus in my recovery. My radiation nurses gave me the superstar award for having washboard abs and not needing assistance in getting off the radiation table each day. We had a good laugh as I've not had washboard abs since being born premature at four pounds, eleven ounces!

I will be released to return home to begin my recuperation period on Friday, May 8, and I look forward to being home! I will not have a final PET scan until roughly three months from now as the radiation and chemo continues to work in the body killing any cells that may be left or mutating. The scan will then determine if I am cancer free. Patience is the key word.

In the meantime, I will be doing regular checks in Iowa City with lab work to determine my progress. It has been a week of ups and downs here. Three of my friends who are also guests here at the Hope Lodge received their "terminal news" this week, sharing that their treatments were not being effective and they were given the options of either continuing treatments or going home to live out their time. All three are fighters and chose to continue the battle.

We talked and prayed together and hopefully, they can fight through the battle as well staying positive through the process. As we talked and prayed, it brought one of my favorite Lance Armstrong quotes to mind, especially after my visit with little Taylor in the Pharmacy.

"If children have the ability to ignore all odds and percentages, then maybe we can all learn from them. When you think about it, what other choice is there but to hope? We have two options, medically and emotionally: give up or fight like Hell."

We all chose the latter and added the spiritual and physical parts of the game plan as well. From an emotional standpoint, I couldn't have done it without my **Home Team**! It will now be my task to mend and prepare for my return to serve as I help you all become the best you can be each and every day. I look forward to that, but will need to stay focused and patient over the next few months as I go through this final stage of the process.

I will be taking an update leave for a while as I move forward following the eighth inning of this contest. I will update you following the game delay when I get the results back from my PET scan toward summer's end. My hope and prayer is to be cancer free and back in the saddle at Holmes Junior High again in the fall.

The score after eight complete innings of play: **Home Team - 8, Visitors - 0!**

An Encouraging Attitude

I plan to **go the distance** by tossing a nine-inning shutout at the **Visiting Team!**

A Spiritual Insight

"Yet in all these things we are more than conquerors
and gain an overwhelming victory through Him
who loved us [so much that He died for us]."[3]
(Paul's encouragement to complete the process and gain the
victory from Romans 8:37)

---

[3] From the Amplified Translation of the Bible

A Step to Consider

Stay focused and patient as you go through the process, no
matter what the challenge!
I've thought how it would be easier to persevere if we knew
exactly where the finish line was, but more often
than not we can't see it.
When I begin to think I've had enough and what I'm working
for isn't going to come to fruition,
I need to hang on just a little while longer.
Focus only on the task that is right in front of me.
When my mind reminds me of all the tasks that follow,
I simply need to bring it back to right here, right now.
No matter what anyone says, just show up and do the work!

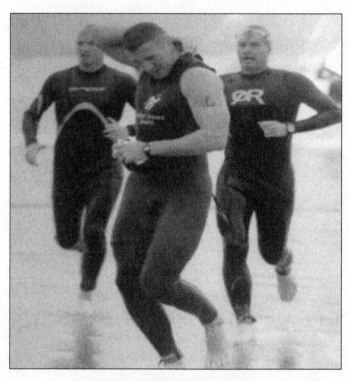

Putting in the Work Pays Off!

Reflection 11

Turning the Negative to the Positive

June 3, 2009

A s I completed my treatment regimen, I felt like a shadow of myself. I am now down sixty-five pounds from the weight I started treatments at. My doctors report that the weight loss is a normal part of the treatment process, however, I have lost a lot of weight in a short period of time and it has affected my strength and stamina. My throat continues to be a concern as I still have difficulty swallowing and speaking, but I hope to make further progress as time goes on.

As my strength and stamina were at an all-time low and a number of side effects from treatments were beginning to surface, my son, John and his fiancé, Shannon began training to compete in a triathlon in San Diego. The rugged training they were both experiencing inspired me to keep up my workout routine despite my declining strength and stamina. A quote that I had read from Michael Jordan also gave me focus to turn that negative into a positive so that ultimately, good results would come for me.

> "I've always believed that if you put in the work, the results will come. Always turn a negative into a positive!" - Michael Jordan

Yet another realization for me was how much I truly missed my students and staff during my time away. The saying that "sometimes you don't know how much something means to you until you don't have it" really rang true for me. I couldn't wait to return to work to be a part of their lives, but first I had to take the time to mend physically and emotionally. I plan to return to work this summer as my energy and stamina allow so that I can be fully operational to return to Holmes in the fall!

I had an appointment with my Oncologist on Monday and my lab work showed that my blood counts have changed some since finishing treatments and some side effects of the treatments will need to be addressed. The tumors in my throat have shrunk, however, there still appears to be a soft tissue mass. Our hope is that the radiation and chemo will continue to work on that mass and eliminate it. If not, I may need to have some surgery done to eliminate it.

I have a number of appointments over the summer with the big one being my PET scan the first week in August to determine if treatments have been successful in helping me become cancer free. I am approaching that date with a positive attitude and need you to know that I could not have successfully made it this far without all of your notes, letters, cards, and kind acts.

An Encouraging Attitude

My plan is to prepare over the summer for a positive year
starting next fall!
Refuse to grow discouraged by communing with God
who provides us the nutrients to grow the strength and
courage to make it through!

A Spiritual Insight

"My only aim is to finish the race and complete the task the
Lord Jesus has given me
—the task of testifying to the good news of God's grace."
(Paul as he focuses on completing what the Lord called him
to do in Acts 20:24)

A Step to Consider

Always turn a negative into a positive!
Remember, "This is the beginning of a new day. I can waste
it or use it for good.
What I do today is important because I am exchanging a day
of my life for it. When tomorrow comes, this day
will be gone forever,
leaving in its place something I have traded for it.
I want it to be a gain, not a loss; good, not evil;
success, not failure—
in order that I shall not regret the price I paid for it today." -
Author Unknown

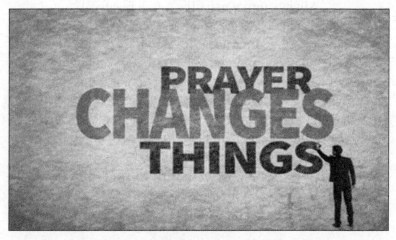

"Be joyful in hope, patient in affliction, faithful in prayer." –
Romans 12:12

Reflection 12

Ninth Inning Shutout!

August 9, 2009

As I anxiously awaited the PET scan, I began experiencing some pitfalls shortly after being released from Iowa City. Now, more than ever, I needed to lean on the connections I had made during treatments to keep my mind, body, and spirit in survival mode.

One of the connections that was truly enhanced by this experience was my relationship with God. God gave us the Bible to teach us about ourselves and to help handle some of life's big challenges. This contest certainly was one of my life's big challenges. As I read His word, it became almost like when I got my first cell phone. I never missed the phone until I got one. The Bible and prayer became much the same for me. I began reading and finding the support and love I needed from God to go along with all the connections I had made with others on my journey. Prayer and my relationship with God continued to grow stronger during the hard times that I had weathered since being diagnosed.

Then the Lord blessed me with some good news! My PET scan on August 4 showed that the cancer cells in my body appear to be dead! As of today, I am cancer free and a survivor!

My doctors were as thrilled as I was about the results and I thank God every day for their expertise and compassionate demeanor. This summer has been a difficult one as I have been battling some side effects following my cancer treatments and did have to have surgery on July 28 to help correct some of the issues. Initially, the surgery did not appear to be successful, but following a checkup last Thursday, I am slowly making some progress.

I'm praying that things continue to improve and that I can get back to a normal routine while regaining some strength and stamina before school starts. I am anxious to get back to work and rededicate myself to serving the needs of our young people here in Cedar Falls. I have certainly missed them during my time away.

We extend our most humble and sincere thanks to our **Home Team**. You have helped me toss a shutout against this formidable foe.

Final score **Home Team - 9, Visiting Team - 0!**

An Encouraging Attitude

The Lord blessed me with some good news.
My PET scan showed I am cancer free and a cancer survivor!
I have felt God's peace as a gift and plan to open that gift by sitting quietly with Him
and placing my trust in Him in every area of my life.

A Spiritual Insight

"All Scripture is God-breathed and is useful for teaching, rebuking, correcting and training in righteousness, so that the servant of God may be thoroughly equipped for every good work."
(2 Timothy 3:16-17)

A Step to Consider

Read God's word and find the support you need for the
journey from God.
God helps us handle the burdens we often carry
by burying them at the foot of the cross with His uncondi-
tional love for us.
That love can free us from fear, anger, anxieties, and the troubles we face in this life.

Part III: Important Connections

The Journey Continues...
2010

My first anniversary since being diagnosed with cancer was certainly an emotional time for me. As my reading continued, I found great comfort in a book recommended by a good friend who had provided me guidance throughout my treatments. The book was titled, *The Last Lecture,* written by Professor Randy Pausch. It is Randy's story of being diagnosed with an aggressive form of pancreatic cancer and given three-six months to live. He developed a "Last Lecture" designed to tell his story to his three young children, the oldest of which was only five. Randy's book was truly inspiring for me.

Trust in my doctors and the hope that God would help carry me through this challenge had been a focus for me over the past year. Hope had provided me a solid foundation in the present, while God had provided me with a healthy dose of joy and peace during those challenging times. I tried hard not to dwell on what had gone wrong along the way, but rather focus on what to do next, spending my time and energy moving forward to find solutions to the challenges.

Prayer allowed me to go inside my heart and know myself much better.

I gradually developed a deeper intimacy with God through prayer. My prayer became a conversation, not formal or scripted in any way. God constantly seemed to be guiding me through His word and through the connections I had made along the way. The experience of God's presence through prayer helped me experience Him in everything else—in people, in events, and even in nature.

I recall making an online order to do a phone repair ticket on our landline and a message popped up to move to the next option. It simply said, "ONWARD." It struck me as a great metaphor for the best way to deal with things that don't go the way we planned—a significant health issue, a tough class in which we struggled to keep our students focused, a bad at-bat, or a bad pitch—we need to learn to move "ONWARD."

It reminded me that we shouldn't get stuck in what just happened, but instead let it go and keep moving forward to the next treatment, next class, next at-bat, or next pitch. I continue to pray that when something doesn't go my way, I will let it go and move onward finding a way over, under or around any barrier that stands in my way. I pray as my journey continues, it will continue deepening those precious connections along the way!

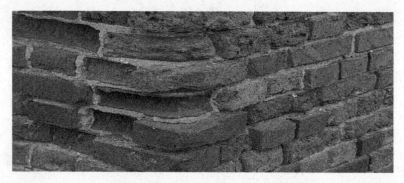
Overcome the Brick Walls of Life

"Live in the present, to enjoy what you have. There are always stumbling blocks in life, or 'brick walls' that you run into. Your task is not to complain about them, but to find ways over, around or through them." - Professor Randy Pausch from his book titled, *The Last Lecture*

Reflection 13

Celebrating Life

March 1, 2010

This has been an emotional weekend for me as I celebrated my birthday and my one-year anniversary of being diagnosed with cancer. There have certainly been some tears over that time, and I have to say that the tear ducts were working well again this weekend. I also have to say they were "tears of joy" as I celebrated life and all it has to offer.

I am happy to report that I remain cancer free following some recent testing in Iowa City as I continue doing regular "maintenance" checks with my team of doctors in Iowa City to monitor things and deal with some treatment side effects. My family and I are excited about that news.

As always, I continue to read and attempt to learn and make sense of things. *The Last Lecture* by Randy Pausch, is a story of a college instructor who was diagnosed with an aggressive form of pancreatic cancer and was given three-six months to live. He developed a "Last Lecture" designed to tell his story to his three young children. His concern was they would not remember him after his passing and he wanted to share what he felt were some of life's important lessons. I have viewed the lecture on YouTube and it is quite powerful. Not surprising, I have connected with Randy and his story. Our journeys have many things in common. I will be reading his book as well, but wanted to share what I felt was his most important message.

> *"Live in the present, to enjoy what you have.*
> *There are always stumbling blocks in life, or*
> *'brick walls' that you run into. Your task is not*
> *to complain about them, but to find ways over,*
> *around or through them. Brick walls are only*
> *there to show how badly we want something,*
> *and they serve to keep those away who aren't*
> *truly committed to achieving their goals. He*
> *asks us to show commitment to your dreams*
> *and goals and not waste your time watching*
> *repeats of TV shows. When your dream is to*
> *develop virtual reality games, become a teacher,*
> *doctor, carpenter, or even run your own busi-*
> *ness, spend your time researching, planning*
> *and heading towards that goal. Don't dismiss*
> *your goals while you spend your extra hours*
> *playing video games. Map out a plan and work*
> *toward your goals."*

You would be very surprised at how many goals are actually within reach if you focus on them. Yes, there will probably be some failures along the way, but just remember, failure equips us to value learning over the appearance of smartness, and to relish challenge and effort while using those errors as routes to mastery.

Over the past year, I have learned that life is truly an adventure. As a good friend shared with me this morning, "An abundant life is full of adventure, and it may involve some risks and danger. Don't get stuck and be content to stay put. Step out and enjoy the adventure."

As I celebrated this weekend, I couldn't think of a better way to do that than by standing and watching one hundred sixty-two of my students who were involved in this year's Holmes Spring Show. These students and their directors worked so hard to put on such a great show, and I can't begin to tell them how proud I am of all of them. For me, that was an adventure worth remembering! They all have been a blessing to me throughout this entire contest and I will continue to serve them and their needs, helping each of them reach their individual dreams and goals. I truly look forward to many more adventures with all of them!

I have listed the link to Randy Pausch's "Last Lecture" for those who may be interested in viewing it. http://www.youtube.com/watch?v=ji5_MqicxSo.

An Encouraging Attitude

Failure equips us to value learning over the
appearance of smartness,
and to relish challenge and effort while using those
errors as routes to mastery.

A Spiritual Insight

"The thief comes only in order to steal and kill and destroy.
I came that they may have *and* enjoy life,
and have it in abundance [to the full, till it overflows]."[4]
(Jesus in John 10:10)

A Step to Consider

An abundant life is full of adventure and it may
involve some risks and danger.
Don't get stuck and be content to stay put. Step
out and enjoy the adventure.

---

[4] Taken from The Amplified Translation of the Bible

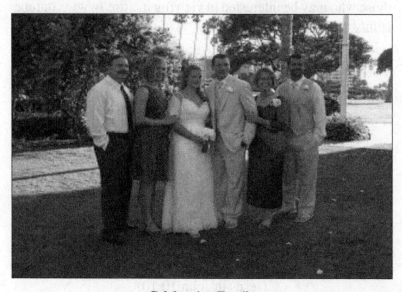

Celebrating Family

Reflection 14

The Right Mental Attitude

March 27, 2010

J ust over a year has passed since I was diagnosed, and I still have a difficult time verbalizing my journey. The "pesky" side effects of treatments have become a part of my daily existence. My **Home Team** doctors have been providing me with some options to help deal with them.

I felt blessed to have had the opportunity to spend another Easter with my family, which had grown since my son John's wife Shannon joined our family last fall. As part of Lenten season, my pastor asked if I would be willing to share my journey with the congregation as a part of his series entitled, "The Way of Anticipation." I had to give that some thought, as I wasn't sure I could stand in front of everyone and share my journey without breaking up emotionally. I've never been shy about presenting, but this was different. My heart, mind, and voice filled with emotion when I verbally attempted recalling parts of the journey.

After praying long and hard about it, I decided to share my journey with our congregation and prayed that God and Pastor Brian would have my back if I emotionally broke down while presenting. My purpose was to provide some hope to those who may be facing a similar journey. My mindset revolved around having a grateful attitude no matter what my circumstance. Just as my battle to defeat cancer had a lot to do with attitude, so did this opportunity to share.

My hope is that it will encourage them to take the opportunity to be open about their struggles and seek out their friends as a means of support to provide them hope and comfort as well. I have placed the links to my message below. I have titled it: *Reflections from the "Home Team"...Go the Distance* (http:// vimeo.com/53873087).

Being a former history teacher, I remembered a quote from Thomas Jefferson that comes to mind frequently for me when thinking about attitude.

> **"Nothing can stop the man with the right mental attitude from achieving his goal; nothing on earth can help the man with the wrong mental attitude."**

Seems pretty simple, but I tend to stumble over it almost every day. It was time to develop a positive mindset about sharing my journey.

I had some surgery a couple weeks ago to deal with some treatment side effects and am happy to share that I still remain cancer free following a series of tests in Iowa City. We are all excited about that news! I have had a consultation with my doctors in Iowa City and have been given a treatment plan that will involve Hyperbaric Oxygen (HBO) treatments to help assist healing some of the damage done in my neck and throat from radiation.

That will involve thirty dive tank treatments, which I plan to begin once school is out this summer. My doctors feel the treatments will give me the best opportunity for long term healing benefits. I will need to clear my next PET scan, however, in May before beginning as the oxygen treatments can actually

stimulate cancer cell growth if any cancer cells are still present.
I look forward to moving ahead with that plan!

An Encouraging Attitude

**"Nothing can stop the man with the right mental attitude
from achieving his goal;
nothing on earth can help the man with the wrong mental
attitude." – Thomas Jefferson**

A Spiritual Insight

"They triumphed over [their enemy]
by the blood of the Lamb and by the word of their testimony."
(Apostle John's encouragement from Revelation 12:11)

A Step to Consider

Be open about your struggles.
Seek out friends as a means of support
to provide hope and comfort.

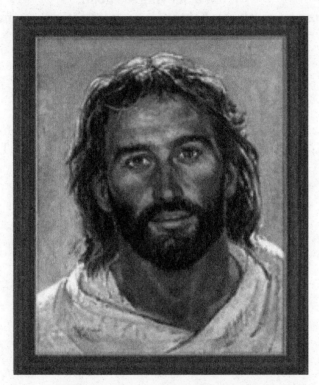

"Smiling Jesus" painted by Frances Hook

Reflection 15

God Never Blinks

May 20, 2010

As I thought about what my future might hold given some of the physical and emotional issues I have been having, I questioned why God was not showing me what was on the road ahead. However, I have chosen to put my trust in Him, praying that He would equip me for the journey if I simply stay in touch with Him. His presence in my life has become my best roadmap!

Spending that special time with Him in the Scriptures each day was refreshing, and provided me a personal "inner experience" feeling God actively and lovingly working in my life. I felt more confident facing each day by simply starting it with Him, allowing His Word to guide my path.

My reading continued as a friend had suggested a book by Regina Brett titled, *God Never Blinks*. As I began reading it, it took me back to a retreat I had as a senior in High School called Teens Encounter Christ (TEC). I was given a picture of a "Smiling Jesus" painted by Frances Hook at that retreat. I have carried that image with me ever since. In that picture, Christ's face glows with peace and a sense of calm. I have included that picture as this reflection's image as it depicts for me the unfailing love that Jesus has for me in all circumstances.

It provides me a sense of calmness no matter what hardships I face. He is always there, "never blinking" at the challenges I am presented. That thought and image has helped carry me through some extremely difficult times.

Regina Brett also has a wonderful piece called, *50 Lessons for Life's Little Detours*. I've attached a link to her YouTube presentation. Both are a good read and I recommend them.

Link to 50 Lessons for Life's Little Detours
http://www.youtube.com/
watch?v=_4hJSE8_wsw&feature=related

I wanted to share some good news, too. I spent Tuesday in Iowa City doing follow up testing and am happy to report my PET scan showed no cancer cells at this time and my blood count is now in the normal range so I am able to discontinue my anti-viral meds! I'm getting closer to prescription free, which is one of my goals! My throat still has inflammation and swelling from the radiation, however, my doctors feel that the hyperbaric oxygen treatments I will be undergoing this summer will help heal that concern. I will be going through thirty consecutive sessions at two hours per day and hope to begin as school ends in early June. I am hopeful healing occurs quickly as well.

An Encouraging Attitude

Christ's face glows with peace and a sense of calm and
depicts for me the unfailing love in all circumstances.
He is always there, "never blinking" at the challenges I am
presented
and has helped carry me through some extremely difficult times.

A Spiritual Insight

"Love never fails.
And now these three remain: faith, hope and love.
But the greatest of these is love."
(Promise from God in 1 Corinthians 13:8, 13)

A Step to Consider

Spend time with God in the Scriptures each day and feel Him actively and lovingly working in your life.

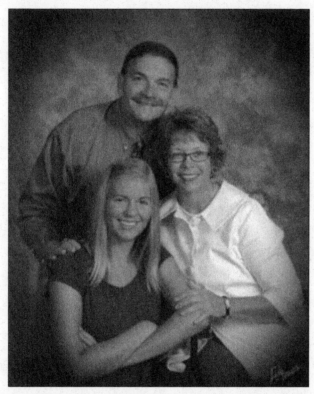

"Keep yourself busy with the things in life that depend on you."

Reflection 16

Building Positive People

August 21, 2010

Tests indicate I'm still cancer free and I'm excited about that news as you can well imagine. I spent sixty hours in a Hyperbaric Oxygen chamber this summer mending from the side effects of radiation and chemotherapy at Mercy Hospital in Cedar Rapids. Once again, I have had excellent caregivers who have made the experience such a positive one. I had to have ear tubes placed in my ears early on during treatments due to pressure during the dives. I survived that and have finally completed my thirtieth and final dive, so I am seeing the light at the end of the tunnel and it looks pretty positive.

I had surgery on July 23, at which time I had dental implant posts drilled into my jaw so that I could have my molars back which were removed prior to radiation treatments last spring as a precaution. My surgeon was a great guy who I affectionately referred to as "Bob the Builder." He worked in my mouth with drill bits and ratchets while implanting the posts into my jaw. I decided to stay awake throughout the process given potential concerns with anesthesia. Dr. "Bob," as I affectionately referred to him, even offered to place a sticker on my forehead to show his appreciation for being a good patient. My kind of guy! Other than looking like "Jabba the Hut" for a day or two after surgery, I came out of it pretty well. I will need to heal for the next three months at which point I can have my molar implants attached! No more oatmeal and cottage cheese!

As Randy Pausch shared in his book, *Last Lecture,* "We cannot change the cards we are dealt, just how we play the hand." I'm looking for a hand that includes some solid food and a chance to once again taste things! Oh, the little things that we often take for granted can become so very special.

At times, I was feeling pretty lousy and began wondering the cause of what was making me feel so lousy. As all those negative thoughts began to enter my mind, I paused and reminded myself I can't argue with reality. When I argue with reality, I generally lose. I began to realize that I couldn't rely on my body always feeling the way I want it to in order for me to be happy and pain free. If I did, I'd be wasting a lot of time and emotion. Not in my control, so I placed trust in my doctors and God to help put this time behind me.

Our time in this life is limited and none of us knows when it will be over. So, it made sense to decide that I would enjoy each day, no matter what. At the very least, I wanted to take a neutral attitude towards the things I couldn't control.

My reading took me to Steve Siemens who owns and operates the "Building Positive People" Corporation based in West Des Moines. He makes a great point in asking, "Why worry about the things you can't control, when you can keep yourself busy controlling the things that depend on you?" *90 Minutes in Heaven* by Don Piper has also provided me with some wonderful guidance over the summer. In it, Don shares ninety readings that address the everyday hardships everyone endures while offering suggestions on how to find serenity in dealing with life's trials.

School starts on August 25, and I have been busy getting ready to kick off yet another year feeling blessed to be able to be back working with a group of students and staff that I truly love. I continue to read and have incorporated some thoughts into my opening presentation to students and staff from Steve Siemens.

"You can't control the length of your life, but you can control its width and depth. You can't control the contour of your face, but you can control its expression. You can't control the weather, but you can control the atmosphere of your mind. Why worry about the things you can't control, when you can keep yourself busy controlling the things that depend on you?"

I plan to keep myself busy this year with the things in my life that depend on me. My family, my students, and my staff at Holmes Junior High will be my focus as the school year begins.

An Encouraging Attitude

I decided I would enjoy each day, no matter what.
I wanted to take a neutral attitude towards the things I couldn't control.

A Spiritual Insight

"Whoever dwells in the shelter of the Most High
will rest in the shadow of the Almighty.
I will say of the LORD, He is my refuge and my fortress,
my God, in whom I trust."
(David as he teaches us to deal with life's issues in
Psalm 91:1-2

A Step to Consider

Be filled with God's peace and joy
as you overcome the obstacles you face in your daily life
while seizing every moment to live life to its fullest!

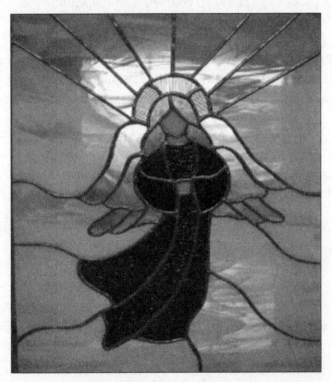

My Guardian Angel "Angelina"

Reflection 17

Adjust and Move On

November 14, 2010

L ate summer and early fall presented a number of challenges for me. The cancer cells remained in remission, but now I had to deal with the troublesome side effects I had been warned about following treatments.

I began using much of my energy wondering about what was on the road ahead. When faced with difficult situations and choices, my mind often tended to click into overdrive. That is when I needed to remind myself to have confidence in God, trusting He will not forsake me in my time of need.

I also realized that if I indulged in worries, pain, and anxieties they could quickly turn into idols. I began to break free from them by trusting and refreshing myself in God's word and letting Him into my heart. God doesn't expect perfection, it's our effort that pleases Him. I was making the effort by beginning each day connecting with Him through prayer and reading scripture.

I have to admit, the side effects of treatments often took over my thinking, and it was easy to indulge them. Perseverance became a daily part of my existence. That is when I began to lean on my precious **Home Team**. With their help, I began to feel more alive, more awake, and more ready to take on the challenges.

"I needed that boost given some of the other stuff going on, and I think it was my Guardian Angel whom I affectionately refer to as Angelina, awakening my heart yet again."

I traveled to see my team of doctors in Iowa City last week for my three-month checkup and my lab tests still show no cancer cells. I'm elated about that news. I have been battling the ongoing side effects of radiation and chemo as well as the HBO treatments. However, as one of the interns shared, "You've been through some stuff, but you always seem to find a way to adjust and move on." I thought that was a pretty good analysis of my journey so far. I'm also excited because my three-month healing process from the dental implant posts that were embedded in August will be up on November 29. I have an appointment in Iowa City that day with my dentist to have new molar implants put in!

I'm hoping at long last to feel like my old self again. I'm also trying to decide what my first "chewy meal" will involve. Still up for grabs, but I'm pretty sure it won't include cottage cheese or applesauce! I've also had some issues with my hearing following treatments as the radiation, chemo, and HBO did a number on my auditory system. I'm working through that now and will make the adjustments I need to make with some hearing assistance. Tricia has said I've had a problem with that for a number of years, but little did she know that was just selective hearing when it came to "Honey Do" lists. Now I may have a legitimate reason to not hear some of those requests, but it sure feels great to be able to tackle all those duties again.

School has kept me busy and has tested my stamina and endurance. So far I've been able to keep up the pace. I've also continued my morning workouts, which has helped me throughout the whole treatment process. My next trip to Iowa

City will be in February and Dr. "C" is keeping close tabs on my labs. I have another PET scan scheduled at that time, and we will use that scan to evaluate progress.

The past year and a half has certainly given me an opportunity to do a lot of reflecting. Reading has given me new perspectives on many things. A good friend recently sent me a quote from Irish poet and philosopher John O'Donohue that really struck home with me.

> *May the angels in their beauty bless you,*
> *May an angel of awakening stir your heart,*
> *May an angel of healing turn your wounds into*
> *sources of refreshment,*
> *May an angel of compassion open your eyes to*
> *the unseen suffering around you,*
> *And may the angel of death arrive only when*
> *your life is complete,*
> *And you have brought every gift to the threshold*
> *where its infinity can shine.*

I sincerely believe I have met several of those angels in my life so far. Without question, I have developed even more compassion for those suffering from this disease and want to reach out to share a message of hope and strength for those who may be facing similar battles with health issues such as cancer.

I wanted to share how important all of these connections have been in my journey as they provided the strength and courage I needed to fight the fight. That is a very important part of the message of hope I want to communicate. Reaching out to others in my time of need wasn't always easy, but it certainly was necessary! As for that last angel, I'm not quite ready to meet him/her yet as I think I still have some gifts to share with others before my life becomes complete within God's plan for me.

As always seems to be the case in my life when things get a bit tough, I experienced something that brought me back in focus. The past few months have been very challenging, and I want to share an experience I had at a Vocal Concert at school because it really picked up my spirits. I had a little guy approach me as I was handing out programs. He shared his name and that he was eight years old.

I introduced myself and he said, "I know who you are because you and I both have had cancer."

He opened his shirt collar to show me his scars. He had suffered from lymphoma. Kind of took me by surprise. I asked how he was doing and we traded some stories. Then out of the blue he shared that his mom had shared with him my updates that I had posted for students and staff during my treatments. He said those were cool and that he wants to be a principal just like me. I choked up a bit. Once I regained my composure, I asked him to help me hand out programs and greet our con-certgoers. He was quite a helper! He greeted many parents who kept asking who my good assistant was. I shared that he was my new intern who is a principal in training! His chest puffed out and he gave me a big grin.

He then had to introduce me to his mom and brother who is a seventh grader and was singing in the Concert. We had a good visit and he shared that in just four years, he will be a Holmes Tiger and then he can help me every day. I told him I would look forward to that! I needed that boost given some of the other "stuff" going on in my life.

Another good friend delivered a leaded glass angel that I have sitting next to me in my office. That art piece reminds me daily of my Guardian Angel, whom I have affectionately named Angelina. I think she was awakening my heart yet again helping me to realize my **Home Team** was there to help me through this. I have always believed I have a Guardian Angel, and honestly, she has been quite busy in my life covering my back, especially the past couple of years.

If there is one message I want to get to people, it is that when faced with a difficult situation like cancer, or for that matter, any tough situation, it is so important to reach out to others for help and support. The Lord and His angels are always there, but so are friends and family. Be sure to access them.

I have also listed a link to one of my favorite artists, Tommy Emmanuel, who plays my favorite song titled, *"Angelina."* I hope you enjoy it.

Link to: Tommy Emmanuel and "Angelina"
http://www.youtube.com/watch?v=AhR04kmcSXU

An Encouraging Attitude

If there is one message I want to get to people,
it is that when faced with a difficult situation like cancer or
any tough situation,
it is so important to reach out to others for help and support.

A Spiritual Insight

Romans 5:3 states, "Suffering produces perseverance."

A Step to Consider

The Lord and His angels are always there,
but so are friends and family.
Be sure to access them.

The Journey Continues...
2011

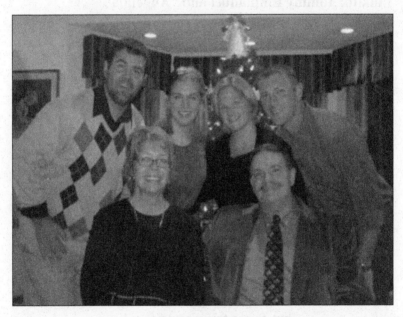

My "Home" Team

Reflection 18

Spring Training

February 13, 2011

As I anxiously awaited my next appointments in Iowa City, I continued to focus on the importance of taking some quiet time each day to sit in stillness to reflect and experience God's unfailing love for me. I needed the certainty of His loving presence to weather the physical and emotional storms that were now confronting me.

Being completely honest, sometimes life just seems hard and discouraging. The challenges we face can be major and life altering, or they can be a series of little things that begin to pile up on us. My goal of being cancer free at times seemed just out of reach given some of the reports and symptoms I was experiencing. Frustration was beginning to dominate my thoughts.

As that happened, I needed to find a way to keep moving forward. I had to find a way to take another step, dig deeper, and believe that things would get better. Often with health issues, that process can be a lost art. I recalled being discouraged in the past, but I have always seemed to find a way to persevere. Reaching out to others when I've needed assistance or encouragement has been especially helpful. I made a commitment to myself to get through it with the help of my **Home Team** — one day and one step at a time.

I wanted to update you as my second anniversary of being diagnosed with cancer approaches. I have spent considerable time in Iowa City this past week working through some concerns with my team of doctors. Lots to think and pray about. I have been working through an infection in my system and my labs have been irregular since December's checkups. My white cell count is extremely low, and my oncologist discussed a number of reasons as to why that may be. His concern is that the **Visiting Team** may be back attacking my white blood cells.

He plans to have me back in Iowa City on Wednesday, February 23, to do another series of labs to recheck my white cell count and do a bone marrow biopsy (where the white cells are produced). That will determine if cancer has returned. We are hopeful there may be another explanation. The journey has been like a roller coaster, with many ups and downs, but I know there is a plan, and I'm preparing myself physically, emotionally, and spiritually if I have to go extra-innings with the **Visiting Team**. How ironic that this is happening as pitchers and catchers report for spring training. I am thankful that my bullpen is in place, ready to go if needed.

I often think of Randy Pausch's comment in his book, *The Last Lecture*, and I keep telling myself "no matter what tomorrow brings, today is a wonderful day." I need to keep on enjoying it, which is sometimes easier said than done. That is a time when I enjoy reflecting on one of my favorite verses.

Christ is always with us and we can always look forward to the "new" that is to come. I plan to make my two-year anniversary a wonderful day by celebrating with those who have surrounded me with love and support over these past two years!

As I was sitting in Iowa City, thinking about my journey this past week, God walked two people into my life as I was waiting in the cancer treatment center. Sitting to my right was a lovely young mother who was surrounded by her kids, husband, and parents. We struck up a conversation and I learned she had just recently had her leg amputated as a result of cancer.

I was amazed at how upbeat and positive she was. We began talking about how those who surround us such as friends and family help make the journey bearable. Her positive attitude and smile given her difficult circumstance made my concerns dwindle, and I shared with her how much I admired her courage in the battle.

To my left was an inmate sitting in his orange jumpsuit, handcuffed with shackles on his ankles. He had been listening to our conversation. He looked at me after I finished visiting with the young mother and I greeted him as well. I asked how he was doing, and he shared, "I ain't got no one except this deputy." He said he had liver cancer and his survival prospects were not good. He also shared that he lost all those who cared for him long ago due to his drug and alcohol issues. He had used and abused those who loved and cared about him to support his habits. He said there is no doubt that his lifestyle led to him developing cancer as well.

He then shared the infamous line I often hear from former athletes and students, "If I could only do it over." At that point my emotions welled up inside me, which has happened all too often lately. I told him it's never too late to start over. I shared 2 Corinthians 5:17 with him and he shared he wasn't much into the Bible. He did share that he wished he had someone in his life that could have given him some of the love and support the young mother and I had been talking about. I then shared with him that there was someone who cared about him, and all it took was accepting God's love and care for him. I invited him to open a Bible and find out how much God really does care. The deputy then wheeled him into treatment and winked at me, saying he would be sure he provided him with a Bible.

Both these people made me realize yet again how important our friends and loved ones are in helping summon the strength and courage to fight the battle against this disease. I feel so fortunate to have such a team in my dugout! I appreciate your prayers!

"For this reason, since the day we heard about you, we have not stopped praying for you. We continually ask God to fill you with the knowledge of His will through all the wisdom and understanding that the Spirit gives." (Colossians 1:9)

An Encouraging Attitude

"No matter what tomorrow brings, today is a wonderful day." - Randy Pausch

A Spiritual Insight

"Therefore, if anyone is in Christ, the new creation has come: The old has gone, the new is here!"
(2 Corinthians 5:17)

A Step to Consider

Focus on the importance of taking some quiet time each day to sit in stillness to reflect and experience God's unfailing love.

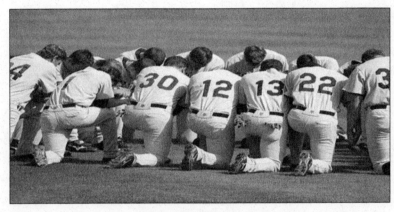

I Have Felt Your Prayers

Reflection 19

Don't Waste Energy on What Cannot be Changed

February 23, 2011

I have tried very hard to focus on being joyful, even when things didn't turn out as I'd hoped. Each day I seemed to be bumping up against things that I didn't want to have happen. I began to realize that God's purpose for me was not to grant my every wish, making my life easy and pain free, but rather to allow me to learn to trust Him in all circumstances. If I was intent on having my way in everything, I soon realized I would be very frustrated most of the time.

Once again I came to understand that God doesn't want us to waste energy regretting things that have happened to us in the past, as they cannot be changed. We have His help in the present and His hope in the future in all that we do. I needed to relax in His presence and trust in His control over my life. I began to feel that presence not only through my prayers, but also through the prayers of others.

I wasn't getting much rest worrying about what my reports in Iowa City might reveal. It became important for me to begin thinking about choosing what I would hold onto and what I would release. Developing that cleansing release thought process can either make you or destroy you. I recall as a hitter in baseball that if I would let the frustration with one at-bat linger, it would end up negatively impacting my at-bats the rest of the game.

I needed to ask myself what it is that I have been carrying around. Is it something that is helping me like a positive belief? If it is, I needed to keep it. But as for past disappointments or frustrations, I needed to try to find a way to let those go, as they'll only drag me down.

Tricia and I returned from Iowa City with some good news. After reviewing test results, Dr. "C" feels that my irregular labs are not due to cancer's return, but rather due to either an infection I've been battling or the strong antibiotics I've been on. Test results show that my white cell count is beginning to rebound which is positive. I have been taken off those strong antibiotics and my doctors will be monitoring my progress without them to see if I can manage to continue to improve. Still some abnormalities, (I've always had those), but at this point, the **Visiting Team** has not returned to my dugout!

I have felt my **Home Team's** prayers and support over the past two weeks and I want you to know it is a powerful thing to experience, and I sincerely thank them all!

Pastor Blaine Schmidt talks about how conversations with people we are close to are to be valued. As we chat, laugh, cry, tell stories of joy and pain, and sit for hours, we often say, where did the time go? We value these ongoing relationships, and we should. I know they have helped me along my journey!

Many of us pray with a wish list of wants. When we develop a relationship with God, like we do people, we can grow into the place of having prayer time that ends with asking, where did the time go?

An Encouraging Attitude

I began to realize that God's purpose for me was not to grant
my every wish,
making my life easy and pain free,
but rather to allow me to learn to trust Him in all
circumstances.

A Spiritual Insight

"God is our refuge and strength,
an ever-present help in trouble."
(Psalm 46:1)

A Step to Consider

God doesn't want us to waste energy regretting things
that have happened to us in the past, as they cannot be changed.
We have His help in the present and His hope in the future
in all that we do.

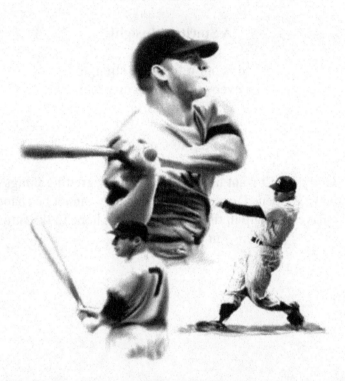

Mickey Mantle – "We admired him for not taking the easy way out."

Reflection 20

Don't Take the Easy Way Out

April 17, 2011

S pring had arrived and baseball was on my mind. No matter how much my spirits fell due to the frustrating side effects of treatments, the dawn of a new season gave me something positive to look forward to. Part of that positivity included developing a grateful mindset no matter what came my way.

For me, this became more difficult as those burdensome health issues continued to appear following treatments. I found that with a grateful heart, even when dealing with those issues, blessings I may never have understood or experienced seemed to come my way. I know this was partially due to God's loving presence and care for me, which always helped brighten my vision of life. I also found this to be true of my supportive close friends, who helped make those difficult times bearable.

I took a lesson from one of my childhood idols, Mickey Mantle, as well as some encouraging words from one of my pastors about not taking the easy way out in life. Both messages came at just the right time for me and provided me some inspiration in playing through the physical and emotional challenges that life had dealt me.

There is something about the crisp crack of baseball bats, scattering line drives, and the smell of fresh, green grass in the spring that just makes me smile. I have had some recent testing in Iowa City and still remain cancer free as I move toward celebrating my second Easter season since being diagnosed.

My recent tests centered on the hearing loss I have sustained following treatments. It appears that I will be able to get some hearing assistance to restore some of the loss. I'm working on that now with my team of doctors in Iowa City. That is great news, except I won't be able to use the standard line of "I didn't hear that" with Tricia any longer when it comes to completing my "To Do" list. I'm also fighting a pesky infection without the use of antibiotics while my white cell count continues to be on the rise. That is good news.

I have been reading and reflecting on some of the support and messages I have been receiving from many people over the past few weeks. It all came together for me this morning as I reflected on a message I heard from Pastor Dennis at services today. His focus was on not taking the easy way out. Ironically, I received an email from a good friend about a week ago sharing the eulogy of Mickey Mantle, one of my childhood heroes. As Pastor Dennis shared his message this morning, some powerful thoughts stuck with me as I reflected on Mickey's eulogy, which was delivered by Bob Costas.

> *"In the last year, Mickey Mantle, always so hard on himself, finally came to accept and appreciate that distinction between a role model and a hero. The first he often was not, the second he always will be. In the end, people got it. And Mickey Mantle got from America something other than misplaced and mindless celebrity worship. He got something far more meaningful. He got love -- love for what he had been; love for what he made us feel; love for the humanity and sweetness that was always there mixed in*

with the flaws and all the pain that wracked his body and his soul."

"We knew he played when he was hurt, and we admired him for not 'taking the easy way out' and asking for days off, the way players would today."

The "Mick" played through many of the physical ailments that racked his body while he continued to play, winning the hearts and souls of baseball fans everywhere. He didn't take the easy way out and always seemed to stay in control and be upbeat, despite the suffering he was going through. That was one of the reasons I so admired him as a young player myself.

There seemed to me to be a lot of parallels for those who face the challenges of a cancer diagnosis and subsequent treatment and recovery as we do our best to continue a life of service to others. Life often sends us challenges that we have to play through. Just as Mickey made organ donation his ninth inning rally cry, we each need to find a way to serve others in a meaningful way in our lives, and not take the easy way out. I've listed a link to Mickey Mantle's eulogy below if you are interested in reading it.

Eulogy of Mickey Mantle: http://jerry.praxisiimath.com/the_mick.html

Jesus didn't take the easy way out either when faced with fulfilling His Father's promise to us. He stayed in control, using courage and conviction to face the suffering. He endured knowing a new life would emerge for us through His Resurrection.

I also wanted to share a quote by Jackie Robinson, yet another of my heroes, as well as a video clip about unselfishly serving others sent by another friend which has really struck home with me this week. Jackie's quote reads: "A life is not important except in the impact it has on other lives."

Despite the physical and emotional struggles we all face on a regular basis, we can choose not to take the easy way out by unselfishly serving others using the gifts we have each been given. A wonderful example of that can be found in the clip below titled *"Gesto de amor."*
https://www.youtube.com/watch?v=Qx1oAImbDnE

An Encouraging Attitude

Jesus didn't take the easy way out when faced with fulfilling
His Father's promise to us.
He stayed in control, using courage and conviction to face
the suffering.
He endured for each of us knowing a new life would emerge
through His Resurrection.

A Spiritual Insight

"Fixing our eyes on Jesus...
For the joy set before him, he endured the cross, scorning
its shame,
and sat down at the right hand of the throne of God.
Consider him who endured such opposition from sinners,
so that you will not grow weary and lose heart."
(Hebrews 12:2-3)

A Step to Consider

Despite the physical and emotional struggles we all face
on a regular basis,
we can choose not to take the easy way out
by unselfishly serving others using the gifts we have
each been given.

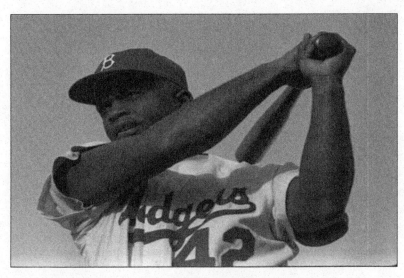

Jackie Robinson – "You can spend your time complaining *or* by playing the game hard."

Reflection 21

Working Hard to Achieve Goals

September 19, 2011

A s fall rolled around, I continued to put a lot of hard work in maintaining the physical and emotional gains I had made following treatments. I began to realize that the greatest thing to come out of all the hard work wasn't necessarily what I got for it, but rather what I had become for it. Hard work doesn't always guarantee you will accomplish everything you set out to do. Life tends to throw us curves and there are plenty of factors that are outside of our control.

Sometimes despite our best efforts, we don't get the results we want. The good news is that while results aren't always what we are shooting for, the most important thing is who we become by working hard to achieve our goals.

I often think back to the work involved with my fellow patients at Hope Lodge who were also battling cancer. The results weren't always what they were hoping for. When focused on process, making life about developing good work habits and a positive mindset rather than an end result, we can gain the strength and courage needed to help carry us through the challenges we face.

My reading took me back to a quote from Randy Pausch about Jackie Robinson. Jackie provided me such a powerful role model, showing how a strong work ethic and positive mindset could carry you through even the most difficult challenges. Jackie couldn't face the challenges of breaking the color barrier in baseball without support, and I couldn't have faced my challenges battling cancer without support. My **Home Team** provided that support for me, and even though cancer had invaded my body, I would never let it invade my soul!

There have been a few bumps in the road over the past month or so. I have been dealing with jaw pain that has been there for some time along with difficulty swallowing given some inflammation and soreness in my throat. The pain has been pretty persistent and not improved. Tricia won't acknowledge she has been punching me or choking me in my sleep, so I thought I'd better get down to my doctors in Iowa City and have things checked.

After not improving for the past few weeks, my concern was that the cancer had returned, which has been a regular part of my roller coaster ride since the spring of 2009. I had a pretty thorough checkup along with some reconstruction work done in my throat Friday. The good news is the cancer has not returned. Other than having a voice that sounds like Luca Brasi (of Godfather fame) and having a tender throat, I'm doing okay and getting some energy back.

I've had quite a bit of time to reflect on some things, and as usual, a message at our Sunday service this past week helped put things back in in perspective for me. A series called, "Family Matters" has been focusing on Genesis and Ephesians and the fact that God observed, "It is not good that man should be alone." That is why He created and established the gifts of marriage, family, and community in His image.

I have come to realize the importance of these gifts as they offer the hope and promise of restoration and new life no matter what the world brings your way. Even though cancer invaded my body in the spring of 2009, it will **never invade my soul!** My family, friends, and community have provided me with the support that has enabled me to make it thus far, and I truly appreciate the fact that they continue to shape and nurture my journey with cancer.

As Randy Pausch said in his book, *The Last Lecture,* while referring to Jackie Robinson:

> "Don't complain, just work harder. It was in his contract not to complain, even when the fans spit on him. You can spend it complaining or playing the game hard. The latter is likely to be more effective."

An Encouraging Attitude

Even though cancer invaded my body in the spring of 2009, I would never let it invade my soul!

A Spiritual Insight

"Come to me, all you who are weary and burdened, and I will give you rest. Take my yoke upon you and learn from me, for I am gentle and humble in heart, and you will find rest for your souls. For my yoke is easy and my burden is light." (Jesus in Matthew 11:28-30)

A Step to Consider

Continue to play the game hard no matter what cards you are dealt, and continue to rely on those who are close to you for support along the way.

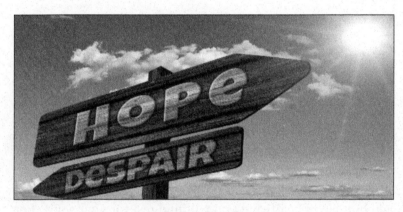

A Path to Freedom

Reflection 22

Minimizing Worry and Maximizing Positivity

December 10, 2011

A s the side effects of radiation and chemo persisted, my
mindset was regularly sidetracked. Worry about those
physical issues continued to be as much a battle for me as the
side effects themselves. A good friend shared with me a definition of worry that made sense to me as I tried to manage my
thoughts. It was a simple thought that provided me some clarity.

**Worry was defined as a matter of thinking
about things at the wrong time.**

I related to that definition as I thought about, or more aptly,
worried about my aches and pains at night as I tried to get to
sleep. That was a problematic because I wasn't getting the rest I
needed for healing to take place. I decided that before I turn out
the lights, if I have worries on my mind, I'd tell myself, **"Not
Now,"** and direct my thinking to other, more positive thoughts.
Sounds simplistic, but it worked for me.

One of my **Home Team** teammates recommended a couple
of books to help embed positive thoughts before resting my

head on my pillow at night. *Nearing Home* by Billy Graham was the first book, which in turn inspired me to read a second book, *Unbroken* by Laura Hillenbrand.

Billy Graham focuses on several things such as: living a life that matters, staying strong despite your circumstances, and most importantly, the hope of Heaven, which are subjects that span all generations and circumstances. He says that the Bible makes it clear that God has a specific reason for keeping us here. He models how we not only learn to cope with the fears and struggles and growing limitations we face as we age, but actually how we can grow stronger inwardly in the midst of these difficulties.

Graham starts out his first chapter using a sports analogy (I always relate to those.). He discusses how he loved baseball and was focused on pursuing it more until God got a hold of his life and changed his direction. The chapter is aptly named, "Running Toward Home." (Sounds kind of familiar doesn't it.) Starting in the first pages and continuing throughout the book, he candidly discusses the hardships associated with aging and the challenges it brings to all. I especially like how he not only describes how to deal with aging, but also how to prepare for it! Some sound advice for all ages.

Unbroken, I just couldn't put down. I found myself dog tired after reading it, having spent much of the night reading, eager to find out whether the story of Louis Zamperini, Olympic runner turned World War II POW, ends in redemption or despair. The following quote made quite an impact on me while Louis and two other POW's faced internment in the Japanese Prison camps:

> *"Though all three men faced the same hardship,*
> *their differing perceptions of it appeared to be*
> *shaping their fates. Louie and Phil's hope dis-*
> *placed their fear and inspired them to work*
> *toward their survival, and each success renewed*

their physical and emotional vigor. Mac's resig-
nation seemed to paralyze him and the less he
participated in their efforts to survive, the more
he slipped. Though he did the least, as the days
passed, it was he who faded the most. Louie and
Phil's optimism, and Mac's hopelessness, was
becoming self-fulfilling."

What a message for anyone who may be facing the ups and downs of a cancer journey, or for that matter, any challenges they may be facing in life. I experienced this back in Iowa City when six of us entered treatments with the same diagnosis and only three of us made it through. Our mindsets of either optimism or hopelessness could most certainly become self-fulfilling!

These books helped me discipline my mind, minimizing worry and maximizing positivity! Each shared different perspectives on dealing with adversity and challenges. They were especially helpful in diverting my mind away from negative thoughts before sleeping. Keeping a positive mindset required much ongoing effort, but I found it a path to freedom from the worries that were a constant presence.

At my regular three month checkup, my lab work and screens revealed what I was expecting for the most part. The aches and pains from the treatment regimen continue with some additional pain I've been experiencing in my upper back. That problem has been intensifying over the past few weeks. It appears that arthritis developing from the radiation treatments in my neck and jaw area has found an additional home in my upper spinal area. The good news is that no cancer cells appeared to be present.

Some treatment options were shared, all of which have additional side effects and I've decided to hold off on them as long as possible and just stick with some anti-inflammatory "stuff" to get through it. I told my doctor that I continue to work out every day, and it's tough to get loose in the mornings, but once I get going, it seems to dissipate a bit. Guess it's more about mindset than medication at this point. I think the ups and downs of not knowing what may be next are the most difficult part of the journey.

My visits to Iowa City and the opportunities I have had to visit with others who are facing similar challenges always brings to mind Regina Brett's quote in *God Never Blinks:*

"If we all threw our problems in a pile and saw everyone else's, we'd grab ours back."

Over the past two years, this quote pretty much sums up what I have experienced while visiting with others in the treatment rooms and doctor's offices. Let's take the time to pause and reflect on making a path for Jesus to come into our hearts as we face our daily challenges while allowing our optimism to become self-fulfilling in each of our lives.

An Encouraging Attitude

I decided that before I turn out the lights,
if I have worries on my mind, I'd tell myself, "**Not Now**,"
and direct my thinking to other, more positive thoughts.
Sounds simplistic, but it worked for me.

A Spiritual Insight

"Can any one of you by worrying add a single hour to your life?
Therefore do not worry about tomorrow,
for tomorrow will worry about itself.
Each day has enough trouble of its own."
(Jesus in Matthew 6:27, 34)

A Step to Consider

Keeping a positive mindset requires much ongoing effort, but I found it a path to freedom from the worries that were a constant presence.

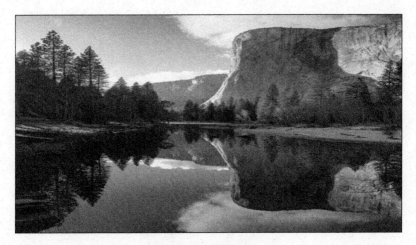

Strength and Peace

The Journey Continues...
2012

Reflection 23

Strength and Peace

February 26, 2012

Over the past several months, I continued to experience times of weakness. My health, worries about the future, and my need for self-sufficiency began to resurface. I found my mind wandering, trying to think ahead to what my day would include and how I would approach it. I share this because it illustrates how quickly I found myself taken out of the present moment, worrying about a future result that hasn't happened and likely would not happen.

When facing those times of weakness and anxiety, I soon realized that I needed to seek out faith and friends as a means of support. I found it helpful to bring those thoughts to others and to Christ in prayer. I had witnessed a number of people who had withdrawn, and not opened their minds and hearts to others during their time of trial. Lessons of trust often come wrapped in difficulty, but they also bring an opportunity to trust each other even more.

I constantly needed to remind myself to focus on being in the moment, not letting my mind get ahead of itself worrying about my next appointment. Dealing with what I had immediately in front of me, and taking care of my work each day gave me the best chance of having a positive outcome.

I trusted that both God and my **Home Team** would be there always, no matter what.

By beginning each day with that trust, I felt more confident that my story would have a happy ending.

"We often can find God's strength in our times of greatest weakness! My hope is that each of us, as we struggle with whatever those afflictions may be in our lives, will be encouraged to take the opportunity to be open about those struggles and seek out faith and friends as a means of support to provide hope, peace, and comfort.

I am celebrating my three-year anniversary since being diagnosed with cancer in 2009. I am still cancer free and a survivor! My next full scan will come in April and my hope is to get referred to the Survivors Clinic at the University of Iowa's Clinical Cancer Center. The journey continues as I have had some recent tune up and maintenance sessions in Iowa City with regard to some lingering side effects from treatments. I am attempting to manage them through bio-feedback for pain management and daily exercise routines. I am also really trying to continue to avoid the medication route if at all possible and so far it's been working for me.

As my journey continues, I've had several discussions with friends and acquaintances all having a similar connection. Each has had experiences with multiple cancer diagnosis in their families, and all have asked the question "Why has God allowed this to happen to our family?" I have to be honest, that question was one that often came to mind for me during treatments and my journey as well.

As I was sitting in the waiting room in Iowa City earlier this month, a young lady was sitting beside me having a hard time keeping her composure as her husband had been recently diagnosed with a malignant tumor, just after he had lost his father to cancer several weeks earlier. We began to visit, and she shared how she felt overwhelmed at the situation. I shared I was sorry to hear her news, but told her that her husband was in great hands with the team of doctors who work with cancer patients here in Iowa City. Sometimes, listening is the best thing we can do, so I did and offered my prayers for her and her family.

The question this young lady raised is one my family and I have struggled with many times. A comfort for me has been some words that were shared when I was originally diagnosed and working through treatments. "Jesus doesn't save us from something, He saves us for something." These words have provided me a focus over the past three years as I've battled the anxieties and difficulties that go with living through cancer. I truly believe that God cares about our afflictions and is more than able to bring us through them.

We often get placed in what I've heard referred to as the "fiery furnace of testing." Having faith that Christ is with us always can give us the strength and stamina to continue despite those uneasy, painful times we face when battling cancer. I sincerely believe we can have an impact on others who may be facing similar trials by modeling a positive and determined attitude as we battle this disease each and every day. Encouraging others on their journey could be what God is "saving us" for.

The picture included with this reflection is from Yosemite National Park and depicts for me the **strength and peace** that can come from having faith despite the afflictions that can test us. We **can** find God's strength in our times of greatest weakness! My hope is that each of us will take the opportunity to be open about our struggles and seek out faith and friends as a means of support to provide hope, strength, peace, and comfort. I'm truly excited to be able to have the opportunity to celebrate yet another Easter season together!

An Encouraging Attitude

When facing those times of weakness and anxiety,
I realized I needed to seek out faith and friends as a means
of support.

A Spiritual Insight

"Base your happiness on your hope in Christ.
When trials come endure them patiently,
steadfastly maintain the habit of prayer."[5]
(Romans 12:12)

A Step to Consider

Lessons of trust often come wrapped in difficulty,
but they also bring an opportunity to trust each other even more.
Be open about your struggles and seek out faith and friends
as a means of support to provide hope, peace, strength,
and comfort.

---

[5] J.B. Phillips New Testament (**PHILLIPS**) The New Testament in
Modern English by J.B Phillips copyright © 1960, 1972 J. B. Phillips.
Administered by The Archbishops' Council of the Church of England.
Used by Permission.

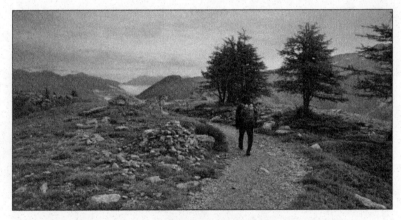

"God doesn't promise us a life full of mountain-top experiences." - Dave Dravecky

Reflection 24

Anger Doesn't Change Circumstances

April 30, 2012

As I moved into spring, I continued to struggle with thoughts and anxieties about my physical symptoms. I was feeling anger about my circumstances when I came across a quote in my reading, which made a lot of sense to me.

"You shouldn't give circumstances the power to rouse anger,
for they don't care at all."
-Marcus Aurelius

That seemed to offer some tough medicine when dealing with our circumstances, but it's certainly true! Circumstances do not change as a result of how angry you get at them. I realized that my feelings resulted from the choices I made. I could choose anger over calm; I could choose fear over courage; I could even choose misery over joy. I decided I needed to determine which choice would be more productive for me.

That is once again when God interjected some people and their thoughts into my life that helped me keep things in perspective. I learned it was a waste of time and breathe getting angry at things that are indifferent to your feelings. It was time to focus on what I could change, on what I could do—not on the angry reaction I was having to my circumstances.

I had my three-month labs and scans done. I've had an upper respiratory problem that has been impacting me for about a month and the side effects of treatments continue to persist. I have been managing those side effects through my biofeedback and daily exercise routines each morning. The thought that my opponent has returned to go extra innings seems to be regularly lurking in my mind. That presents a continuing challenge for me both emotionally and physically.

Several respiratory concerns were addressed by my team of doctors and the good news is that my lungs are clear as the labs and scans have shown that my cancer has not returned. Just as importantly, I have been referred to the **Survivors Clinic!** I will continue to work with my oncologist, Dr. "C", but the rest of my treatments and follow up will be processed through the survivor's clinic on a regular basis until I successfully reach my five-year anniversary. That has been a goal of mine for the past two years, and I'm excited to have nearly reached it!

As so often happens when in Iowa City, I get to visit with people who are experiencing difficult circumstances and I always appreciate the opportunity to interact. As I was sitting in the waiting area between tests today, I had a chance to visit with a young lady who had lost both her legs in a motorcy-cle-car accident about two years ago. As she was riding with her fiancée, a drunk driver hit them while crossing the center-line and her fiancée was killed and she lost both her legs. I was amazed at her upbeat attitude as she talked through the accident. I asked her what she found to be her source of strength as she recovered from the accident. Her reply was simply, "God has always been with me and I'm not alone."

Her positive and upbeat approach while we discussed her accident and the trials that followed inspired and challenged me to remain focused, determined, and positive as I move forward on my own journey. It seems God always puts someone in my life just as I need them to keep me upbeat and moving forward. We shared a prayer together for others in the waiting area who were waiting to be treated and went about our appointments.

I continue to read, finding comfort and inspiration as my journey moves forward. A thought by Fr. Richard Rohr in his book, *Falling Upward,* was very powerful for me.

> "There will always be at least one situation in our lives that we cannot fix, control, explain, change, or even understand... and in turn we learn how to recover from falling by falling."

I've had my share of falls in the past few years and I know that cancer has introduced me to real suffering. In turn, suffering is what has truly strengthened my faith. I need to remain focused, determined, and rely on my faith so that I can recover as I experience those falls. I've also found comfort in reading Dave Dravecy's books, *When you can't Comeback* and *Called Up,* which target the focus, determination, and faith it takes to come back from a journey with cancer.

In his seventh year in Major League Baseball while pitching for the San Francisco Giants, a cancerous tumor was discovered in Dave's pitching arm. The next years were a whirlwind of surgery, radiation, pain, and depression. Eventually, Dave's arm was amputated to stop the spread of the cancer and save his life.

I heard Dave speak a couple years ago at a Fellowship of Christian Athletes rally I attended, and some words he shared that evening have remained embedded in my thoughts.

> "When God wants to do an impossible thing, He takes an impossible man and crushes him."

127

When facing these challenges, our mindset needs to be what Dave talks about during his comeback from cancer surgery to professional baseball.

> "God doesn't promise us a life full of mountain-top experiences. There will be valleys to go through, too. Dark valleys. Disorienting valleys. Valleys of depression and despair. What He promises is not a road map that will give us a detour around those valleys, but that He will walk through those valleys with us. When we emerge from those experiences, we look back and realize that that is where the growth is. It isn't on the mountaintops, above the timberlines; it's in the valleys."

Sometimes it's hard to visualize growth opportunities in the midst of challenges facing us, but that is where our faith, mindset, supportive friends, and family enter the picture.

An Encouraging Attitude

I learned it was a waste of time and breathe getting angry
at things that are indifferent to your feelings.
It was time to focus on what I could change, on what
I could do—
not on the angry reaction I was having to my circumstances.

A Spiritual Insight

"My dear brothers and sisters, take note of this:
Everyone should be quick to listen, slow to speak and slow to become angry,
because human anger does not produce the righteousness that God desires."
(James the brother of Jesus in James 1:19-20)

128

A Step to Consider

Sometimes it's hard to visualize growth opportunities
in the midst of challenges facing us,
but that is where our faith, mindset, supportive friends,
and family enter the picture.

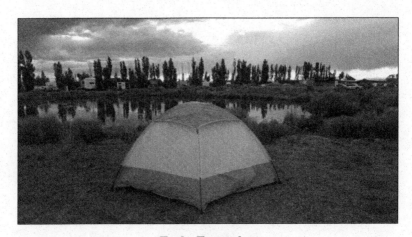

To the Tentmaker

Reflection 25

Ode to the Tentmaker

July 26, 2012

It was now summer, a time my family and I have always used to reenergize. As I had felt the pangs of side effects much of the spring and early summer, some time away at our favorite vacation spot was a welcome and comforting thought. Door County, Wisconsin, has been a favorite of ours for many years.

I've always found peace in nature. When I sit quietly for extended times in nature, I often see that everything changes. Nothing stays in the same shape or form for long. All of the natural world seems to accept the change of seasons. As I think about it, this is so true. As we all age, things just naturally are part of that process for each of us. Hard to accept, but its definitely a reality.

I continue to be cancer free and a determined survivor. I have had some more throat concerns over the past few weeks, but am working through those. They appear yet again to be side effects from chemo and radiation treatments. I continue to successfully manage the arthritis symptoms in my jaw and neck through biofeedback and daily exercise routines each morning. The routine helps keep me motivated to work out each day, which is certainly a good thing.

I have had an opportunity to continue my reading with, *Do Not Lose Heart,* by Dave Dravecky as we spent some time away up in Door County with our family, and that was awesome. We have spent many years traveling to our favorite spot there as a family, camping, biking, swimming, and fishing. It gave me some time to reflect on my journey not only with cancer, but with my family as we have spent all those years camping in tents, trailers, cabins, and more recently vacation homes. If you go camping, you may live in a tent for a few days, you can even make the tent very comfortable. You can bring with you chairs and tables, cookery, and utensils, but you know where you are is still a tent. You would soon need to pack up and go home after camping because a tent is a temporary shelter.

I've always felt it is fun camping in a tent, but it's certainly not home. There is no fireplace, no cozy chair, and no soft bed. It's cold in the winter, hot in the summer, and leaky when it rains. And the older it gets, the more it sags and eventually it frays and tears, kind of like each of us! I have my fortieth High School class reunion coming up this weekend, and I'm guessing I may hear a few stories of sagging, fraying, and tearing which is all part of the maturing process I guess.

In his book, *Do Not Lose Heart,* Dave Dravecky shares a powerful example that illustrates our bodies as temporary tents. The piece reminds me that our focus must be on the building to come which we have with God, not the earthly tent we live in now. The title of the piece is, "O Mr. Tentmaker" and it has provided me a great perspective as I move forward on my journey with this disease.

Writing to the Tentmaker the Tent-Dweller writes:

O Mr. Tentmaker:

It was nice living in this tent when it was strong and secure and the sun was shining and the air warm. But Mr. Tentmaker, it's scary now. You see, my tent is acting like it is not going to hold together; the poles seem weak and they shift with the wind. A couple of stakes have wiggled loose from the sand; and worst of all, the canvas has a rip. It no longer protects me from beating rain or stinging fly. It's scary in here, Mr. Tentmaker.

Last week I went to the repair shop and some repairman tried to patch the rip in my canvas. It didn't help much, though, because the patch pulled away from the edges and now the tear is worse. What troubled me most, Mr. Tentmaker, is that the repairman didn't seem to notice I was still in the tent; he just worked on the canvas while I shivered inside. I cried out once, but no one heard me. I guess my first real question is: Why did you give me such a flimsy tent? I can see by looking around the campground that some of the tents are much stronger and more stable than mine. Why, Mr. Tentmaker, did you pick a tent of such poor quality for me? And even more important, what do you intend to do about it?

In his reply, the Tentmaker writes:

O little tent dweller, as the Creator and Provider of tents, I know all about you and your tent, and I love you both. I made a tent for myself once, and lived in it in your campground. My tent was vulnerable, too, and some vicious attackers ripped it to pieces while I was still in it...on a cross. It was a terrible experience, but you will be glad to know they couldn't hurt me. In fact, the whole experience was a tremendous advantage because it is this very victory over my enemy that frees me to be a present help to you.

O little tent dweller, I am now prepared to come and live in your tent with you, if you'll invite me. You'll learn as we dwell together that real security comes from My being in your tent with you. When the storms come, you can huddle in my arms and I'll hold you. When the canvas rips, we'll go to the repair shop together.

Someday, little tent dweller, someday your tent is going to collapse. You see, I've designed it only for temporary use. But when it does you and I are going to leave together. I promise not to leave before you do. And then, free of all that would hinder or restrict, we will move to our permanent home and together, forever, we will rejoice and be glad.

Dave shares that when we ourselves, a friend, relative, parent or anyone very dear to us is struggling with cancer or some other life-threatening disease, sometimes we feel numbed, bereaved, disappointed, and angry as all kinds of negative sensations flood our minds. We need to remember that though we are suffering the trials of fighting such a battle, it is our earthly tents which are being impacted. We can look forward to forevermore living in a new building, not temporary tents anymore, but rather a new building built by God. There we can live forever and neither death nor suffering will have any sway over us.

An Encouraging Attitude

Though we are suffering the trials, it is our earthly tents
which are being impacted.
We can look forward to forevermore living in a new building
built by God.
There we can live forever and neither death nor suffering
will have any sway over us.

A Spiritual Insight

"For we know that if the earthly tent we live in is destroyed,
we have a building from God, an eternal house in heaven,
not built by human hands."
(2 Corinthians 5:1)

A Step to Consider

Remember we have a God who is with us and
for us in our life's journey.
So refuse to be discouraged along the way and go to Him for
strength and courage.

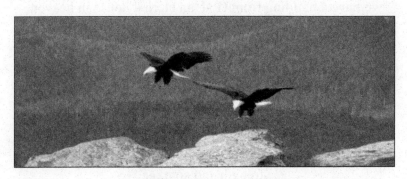

Crows Don't Hang with Eagles

Reflection 26

Crows Don't Hang with Eagles

August 26, 2012

S ummer had provided a refreshing break for me. The fall however began with the loss of several friends and acquaintances. Those losses reminded me of the importance of relationships in my life. One of those friends, just before being involved in a fatal accident had shared, "God knows when we will be born and when we will die, what's in between is up to us."

He was right! God knows everything about us in between, too, and He allows us the freedom to accept His love and guidance along the way. Trusting in Him rather than relying on our own understanding is the most reasonable and joyful way to live. Trusting in family and friends is also a critical piece of any cancer journey.

Side effects of treatments continue to need some attention, and I spent some time in Iowa City recently having testing done regarding some ongoing throat issues. Tests results came back negative for cancer and my doctors suggested some medication to help suppress the treatment side effects. They seem to be working which I am very grateful for. We have also recently had a number of student/parent tragedies in our building involving loss of life, some being cancer related. It has been difficult emotionally to watch people grieve through those losses, just reminding us daily how fragile life really is.

Those recent experiences bring to mind some things that I experienced while undergoing treatments. For me the physical pain experienced from treatments was something I was determined to tolerate, it was the emotional pain of often not knowing what may come next that often ate me up from the inside out. My encouragement to any cancer patient, or for that matter, anyone struggling with emotional pain from suffering or loss is to remember it is important not to ignore the emotional side of suffering. The advice, "Just suck it up" doesn't work.

Our mental state enormously affects our physical state. Fears, grief, and anger all need to be expressed in order to bring physical healing. That is where the power of relationships in healing becomes so important. It is those relationships that can allow us to lean on others; bringing those emotions out in the open to heal. My family and supportive friends have provided that opportunity for me time and again. We need to be there for each other in those times of fear, anxiety, and loss. King David poured his heart out to God in the psalms. We, too, can share those thoughts and feelings with God.

Conventional medical care for cancer has for many years concentrated on destroying tumors without paying much attention to supporting the patient as a whole person. Until recently, most people put themselves in the hands of an oncologist (cancer specialist) and did what they were told. While you almost certainly need a good oncologist to prescribe and monitor your medical treatment, there is often much more to surviving cancer. A well-nourished person with cancer, who is provided with the tools and support to help them maintain their emotional balance, is likely to have a much easier time with cancer and its treatments than a person who is poorly nourished, poorly supported, and stuck in terror and emotional turmoil. A true story a very good friend recently shared with me illustrates just how important emotional support and the power of relationships is in healing. The story comes out of Australia.

FREEDOM and JEFF

Freedom and I have been together eleven years this summer. She came in as a baby American Bald Eagle in 1998 with two broken wings. Her left wing doesn't open all the way even after surgery, it was broken in four places. She's my baby. When Freedom came in she could not stand and both wings were broken. She was emaciated and covered in lice. We made the decision to give her a chance at life, so I took her to the vet's office. From then on, I was always around her. We had her in a huge dog carrier with the top off, and it was loaded up with shredded newspaper for her to lie in. I used to sit and talk to her, urging her to live, to fight; and she would lay there looking at me with those big brown eyes. We also had to tube feed her for weeks. This went on for four-six weeks, and by then she still couldn't stand. It got to the point where the decision was made to euthanize her if she couldn't stand in a week. You know you don't want to cross that line between torture and rehab, and it looked like death was winning.

She was going to be put down that Friday, and I was supposed to come in on that Thursday afternoon. I didn't want to go to the center that Thursday, because I couldn't bear the thought of her being euthanized; but I went anyway, and when I walked in everyone was grinning from ear to ear. I went immediately back to her cage; and there she was, standing on her own, a big beautiful eagle. She was ready to live. I was just about in tears by then. That was a very good day. We knew she could never fly, so the director asked me to glove train her. I got her used to the glove, and then to jesses, and we started doing education programs for schools in western Washington. We wound up in the newspapers, radio (believe it or not) and some TV. Miracle Pets even did a show about us.

In the spring of 2000, I was diagnosed with non-Hodgkin's lymphoma. I had stage three, which is not good (one major organ plus everywhere), so I wound up doing eight months of chemo. Lost the hair - the whole bit. I missed a lot of work. When I felt good enough, I would go to Sarvey and take Freedom out for walks. Freedom would also come to me in my dreams and help me fight the cancer. This happened time and time again. Fast forward to November 2000 the day after Thanksgiving, I went in for my last checkup. I was told that if the cancer was not all gone after 8 rounds of chemo, then my last option was a stem cell transplant. Anyway, they did the tests; and I had to come back Monday for the results. I went in Monday, and I was told that all the cancer was gone.

So the first thing I did was get up to Sarvey and take the big girl out for a walk. It was misty and cold. I went to her flight and jessed her up, and we went out front to the top of the hill. I hadn't said a word to Freedom, but somehow she knew. She looked at me and wrapped both

her wings around me to where I could feel them
pressing in on my back (I was engulfed in eagle
wings), and she touched my nose with her beak
and stared into my eyes, and we just stood there
like that for I don't know how long. That was a
magic moment. We have been soul mates ever
since she came in. This is a very special bird. I
will never forget the honor I have of being so
close to such a magnificent spirit as Freedom.[6]

Cancer is a strange cell. You can go along for years in
remission and then one day it pops its head up again. If you
ever have it, you will never be free of it. Pray for the day there
will be a permanent cure. This brings to mind the importance
of encouraging those around us who may be suffering, just
as Jeff did for Freedom and in turn, Freedom did for Jeff. We
often hear people complaining about their suffering and that
brings to mind a comment made by Joel Osteen which has stuck
with me and seems appropriate after listening to the story of
Freedom and Jeff.

"Encouragement is a wonderful thing, and
people do not receive enough during difficult
times. You need to be around people who are
encouraging. After listening to people gripe
and complain just smile and remember …crows
can't hang with eagles."- Joel Osteen

---

[6] https://www.harpercollins.com/9780062015501/an-eagle-named-
freedom# (Note: As of April 2016 both Freedom the eagle and the author
were still alive and they are considering making a movie of their story.)

An Encouraging Attitude

My encouragement to any cancer patient or anyone struggling with emotional pain,
is remember it is important not to ignore the emotional side
of suffering.
The advice, "Just suck it up" doesn't work.

A Spiritual Insight

"But those who hope in the LORD will renew their strength.
They will soar on wings like eagles;
they will run and not grow weary,
they will walk and not be faint."
(Isaiah 40:31)

A Step to Consider

Just as King David did in the Psalms by pouring his heart
out to God,
we, too, can share those thoughts and feelings with God.

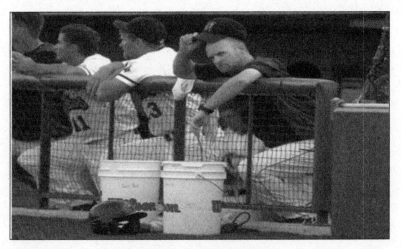

Minor League Thinking

Reflection 27

Minor League Thinking

November 4, 2012

Each day of my journey consisted of 24 hours and every one of them presents unique circumstances for me. Some of those circumstances were painful, both physically and emotionally. Despite that, I seemed to find joy in unexpected places. It required some effort, but by searching for the good and refusing to let my negative responses to them blind me seemed to be the key. It brought to mind a thought shared by one of my nurses during treatments, "Where the heart is willing, it will find a thousand ways, but where it is unwilling it will find a thousand excuses."

As I searched for any good I could find amid my ongoing frustrations, I had the "want to" in my heart, but figuring out the "how to" always seemed a bit more difficult. If I wanted to overcome the frustrations bad enough, I needed to figure out a way how to!

It's been a frustrating couple of months as side effects from treatments have been an ongoing nuisance. I continue to work with my team of doctors in Iowa City adjusting the plan as I move forward. They are a special group of people who continue to work closely with me to help problem solve the aches and pains that accompany the cancer journey. The good news is that the cancer cells continue to appear to be dormant and that is most certainly a positive! There appear to be some issues from treatment that will remain with me including nerve damage and scar tissue from the radiation treatments. They seem to be the culprits in the ongoing aches and pains experienced as a part of each day.

As I often share, these are a very good alternative to having the **Visiting Team** return to my dugout! I will continue to work with the doctors to problem solve these issues and make each day count in making a difference. I continue to read to find comfort and answers to the many questions that enter a person's mind as you ride the roller coaster that each series of tests brings when dealing with those aches and pains. Most recently, I have found comfort and some good old-fashioned common sense in Dave and Jan Dravecky's book, *Do Not Lose Heart*. Of course, it draws an analogy to baseball, so all the more meaningful to me.

> "Sometimes we are tempted to think that life's hardships and setbacks, pain and loss manage to make us think there is no such place as heaven and there is no end to the pain. When thoughts like that begin to bedevil us, we need a dose of 'minor league' thinking. Every minor leaguer knows that, no matter how bumpy and uncomfortable and long the road trip to the next ball field might be, the length of his journey never alters the reality of his destination. The trip won't last forever and the diamond will be waiting for him at the end." - Dave Dravecky

Dave shares that when playing baseball in the Minor Leagues, you had better learn to like busses, because whether you like them or not you are going to see plenty of them. If lucky in the minors, you might get a bus with air conditioning and reclining seats, if not, you may be riding with no shocks and vinyl seats that stick to you like Velcro in the summer heat. I've been there and done that! Either way, the trips from ballpark to ballpark can get long. No matter how long the trip may be, they can always count on one thing: "The length of their journey never alters the reality of their destination." Whether it takes two hours, four hours or ten hours (with a couple of flat tires along the way), he knows he will get there eventually.

That's minor league thinking that results in major league benefits. The point of the trip is to arrive at the destination. No one claims that the long hours spent in an old rundown bus is always pleasant, but what is certain is that the ballpark waits, freshly groomed, and ready to welcome the saints who belong there.

Dave also points out that in the same way, the Bible promises us that no matter how difficult our journey may become, the length of our journey never alters the reality of our destination. Obviously, the Bible is not talking about baseball. Instead, it is talking about the only league that ultimately counts. That is, of course, the one where God is the owner, founder, and commissioner. The stadium is paved with transparent gold, and where all the players are known as saints. It's talking about eternity.

Dave and Jan did a wonderful job of presenting their thoughts while helping me realize that no matter how "bumpy the ride" and even though I may not fully understand His plan, God is preparing me for a far better place than this. It's time for me to implement some "minor league thinking."

An Encouraging Attitude

I needed to realize that no matter how "bumpy the ride" and even though I may not fully understand His plan, God is preparing me for a far better place than this.

A Spiritual Insight

"So we fix our eyes not on what is seen, but on what is unseen, since what is seen is temporary, but what is unseen is eternal." (2 Corinthians 4:18)

A Step to Consider

The length of this journey never alters the reality of our destination.
Minor league thinking results in major league benefits.

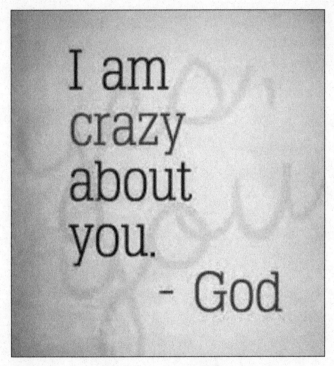

God Is Crazy About You!

The Journey Continues...
2013

Reflection 28

Why did this happen, God?

February 24, 2013

I was nearing my four-year anniversary being diagnosed and had some good news from my **Home Team** of doctors. My labs were beginning to return to their normal ranges, but the question still lingered in my mind as to how God could let this happen to me.

That is when a good friend shared a story reminding me to take charge of my thoughts each day, remembering we will find God when we seek Him above all else. As we face each day's challenges, many thoughts will come and go, and even in the darkest of times, God can brighten our days, blessing us with joy as He puts all things in order in His timing, not ours.

"A daughter is telling her Mother how everything is going wrong, she's failing algebra, her boyfriend broke up with her, and her best friend is moving away. Meanwhile, her Mother is baking a cake and asks her daughter if she would like a snack, and the Daughter says, 'absolutely mom, I love your cake.'

'Here, have some cooking oil,' her Mother offers. 'Yuck' says her daughter. 'How about a couple raw eggs?' 'Gross, Mom!' 'Would you like some flour then? Or maybe baking soda?' 'Mom, those are all yucky!' To which the mother replies: 'Yes, all those things seem bad by themselves, but when they're put together in the right way, they make a wonderfully delicious cake!'

God works the same way. Many times we wonder why He would let us go through such bad and difficult times. But God knows that when He puts these things all in order in His timing, they always work for good! We just have to trust Him, and eventually, they will all make something wonderful!

God is crazy about you. He sends you flowers every spring and a sunrise every morning. Whenever you want to talk, He'll listen. He can live anywhere in the universe, and yet He chose your heart."

May each of you enjoy a slice of that cake as you enjoy those spring flowers and beautiful sunrises each day! God didn't promise days without pain, laughter without sorrow, sun without rain, but He did promise strength for the day, comfort for the tears, and light for the way!

An Encouraging Attitude

God didn't promise days without pain, laughter without sorrow, sun without rain, but He did promise strength for the day, comfort for the tears, and light for the way.

A Spiritual Insight

"But seek first his kingdom and his righteousness, and all these things will be given to you as well." (Jesus in Matthew 6:33)

A Step to Consider

Take charge of your thoughts each day. Remember you will find God when you seek Him above all else.

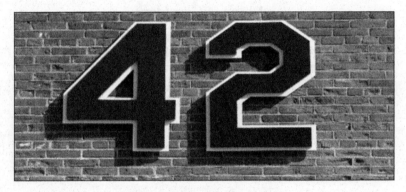

Endurance and Perseverance

Reflection 29

Where Is the Finish Line?

June 1, 2013

Some additional physical concerns began to appear which were indirectly related to treatments and it focused my thoughts on endurance. Over the past four and a half years, it would have been easier to persevere if I had known exactly where the finish line was, but more often than not I couldn't see it.

I recalled reading in Marcus Lutrell's book, *Lone Survivor,* how so many people who enlisted in the Navy Seals training program quit just before the finish line of an exercise because they didn't know they were close to finishing it. When I began to think like I'd had enough and what I was working for wasn't going to come to fruition, I needed to remember to hang on just a little while longer and focus only on the task that was right in front of me. When my thoughts centered on all the tasks that were to follow, I needed simply to bring it back to the here and now.

My blood counts have returned to the normal range, but I've had continued issues with neck and jaw pain as well as some significant hip pain. Long story short, X-rays came back and showed I have a severe case of osteoarthritis and degenerative joint disease in both hips, which seems to have accelerated since treatments. I'll need to have both hips replaced. Guess all those years behind the plate are "catching" up with me.

I'm planning to have the first surgery Tuesday, June 11, and the second surgery done midsummer if no complications arise, so I can get back to enjoying the active life style I have grown accustomed to. The better news is that the cancer remains in check. I was worried that my elevated counts following the virus I had this winter and the increased pains were a signal that the **Visiting Team** may have returned to my dugout. Always seems to be on my mind, so when that happens, I turn to my favorite pastime of reading, particularly about those who have overcome challenges in their lives to make a positive difference for others.

God doesn't waste any pitches when it comes to teaching you about life from the game of baseball! Baseball has taught me many lessons that I have applied to my life, and more importantly, to my relationship with God. I have learned the lesson of endurance from my journey over the past few years. As a good friend recently shared, "hips wear out and can be replaced," and that is a positive way to view this, so I will!

Endurance is defined as the ability to bear pain or hardship, the strength to continue despite fatigue, stress or other adverse conditions.[7] Not sure if the writer of that definition had being a cancer survivor or a Junior High Principal in mind when writing that, but I guess it fits both.

After viewing the recent release of the Movie *"42"* with my wife Tricia, I found it comforting to read all I could find about one of the baseball heroes who had inspired me during my cancer treatments, namely, Jackie Robinson. Talk about endurance, Jackie Robinson was certainly more than an athlete, he was a real man, often standing alone as he challenged and integrated modern Major League Baseball. His task was not easy as he suffered many mental and physical pains along the

---

[7] Merriam-Webster Dictionary© 2017 Merriam-Webster, Incorporated

way. He accepted and overcame the slings, slams, and insults so that young black athletes could dream of playing Major League Baseball.

I struggled in my reading with how he was treated so cruelly by other human beings because of the color of his skin. I don't know of many who could have handled the insults directed his way. One thing that is often not written about or understood about Jackie is that he was a Christian, as was the Brooklyn Dodgers General Manager, Branch Rickey.

When Rickey called Jackie to his office to discuss a contract, he spent three hours grilling Jackie, role playing an insulting fan, a mean spirited player, a snobby hotel manager, a rude head waiter, a condescending sports writer, and a disrespectful teammate (all of which happened during his career). He told Jackie players would come at him with spikes up, throw at his head and that he'd get called out on strikes by racist umpires. When Jackie asked if he was looking for a player who was afraid to fight back, Rickey said, "Robinson, I'm looking for a ballplayer with guts enough not to fight back! You will symbolize a crucial cause, one incident; just one incident will set it back twenty years."

Rickey then reached for a book titled, *The Life of Christ*, written by an Italian priest, Giovanni Papini. Rickey expounded on Jesus' teaching regarding an eye for an eye and a tooth for a tooth by sharing Father Papini's thoughts, "to answer blows with blows, evil deeds with evil deeds is to meet the attacker on his ground. Only he who has conquered himself can conquer his enemies." Rickey closed the book and faced Jackie asking, "Can you do it? I know you are naturally combative, but will you promise that for the first three years in baseball, you will turn the other cheek? Three years, can you do it?" Jackie replied, "Mr. Rickey, I've got two cheeks. If you want to take this gamble, I'll promise you there will be no incidents."

From the beginning, Jackie understood the impact he would make. We will be forever indebted to Jackie Robinson for what he did and for what he endured. There is no doubt in my mind that his faith sustained him, and from that I have learned a great lesson, which has helped carry me on my journey.

It is my hope that my journey can provide some comfort and encouragement for others who may be struggling to endure hardships in their lives, just as Jackie Robinson's journey impacted mine.

Another good friend recently shared the following quote, which has been a powerful reminder to me of how God's plan for each of us works.

"When everything seems like it's falling apart, that's when God is putting things together just the way He wants it!"

I'm sure Jackie Robinson may not have always seen it this way through his experiences at the time, but with reflection, we can certainly see God's plan at work by subjecting Jackie to these abuses during his Major League career and the impact his experience had in helping others achieve their dreams.

An Encouraging Attitude

"When everything seems like it's falling apart,
that's when God is putting things together just the way He wants it!"

A Spiritual Insight

"But in your hearts revere Christ as Lord.
Always be prepared to give an answer to everyone
who asks you to give the reason for the hope that you have.
But do this with gentleness and respect."
(1 Peter 3:15)

A Step to Consider

Remember to hang on just a little while longer.
Focus only on the task that is right in front of you.

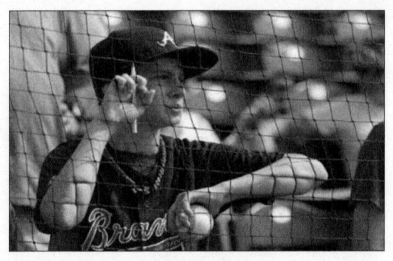

"Be prepared. Luck is truly where preparation meets opportunity." -
Randy Pausch in his book *The Last Lecture*

Reflection 30

Life's Poker Game

August 2, 2013

The anxiety of waiting for results is a normal thing for me, I guess. I knew that I could call upon God to help me find courage and strength as I faced the ongoing issues involving cancer and the side effects of treatments. I continued trying my best to handle them with confidence and determination.

I was experiencing some tough times following the hip replacement I had completed earlier in the summer. A nasty infection had now become the culprit. I am finishing up a third antibiotic and feel this one may have solved the issue. I will be doing some testing early next week to confirm that.

Then while I was in Iowa City on Tuesday to do some cancer lab work, my counts were abnormally high which is a major concern. My team of doctors feels that it could be related to the infection, but wants me back in six weeks to retest. If the counts remain high, I will need to do a series of biopsies to determine if the cancer has returned. As a result, I'm going to hold off having the second hip done until a later date, once fully healed.

I focused on keeping my thoughts away from the negative, but rather concentrated on the strength, peace, and blessings that have come my way through my quiet time with God and the support provided by my **Home Team**.

As Regina Brett shares in one of my favorite books, *God Never Blinks,* "Time heals almost everything. Give time, time." Sometimes it is hard to allow that to play out, however, patience is the key. Regina also shares, "It doesn't matter what has happened to you, it matters what you do with what has happened to you. Life is like a poker game. You don't get to choose the cards you are dealt, but it's entirely up to you how to play the hand."

As often happens in Iowa City, I was waiting yet again in the Cancer Center for results last Tuesday. I closed my eyes to get a little rest, as sleep has been hard to come by as of late. A few minutes passed, and I felt a tap on my shoulder and opened my eyes to once again find little Taylor, (who is not so little anymore). I had met Taylor in the pharmacy during treatments back in April, 2009. He and I had played a game of toss in the pharmacy that day and I had showed him some of my ball tricks.

Taylor and his mom were in Iowa City for their six-month check when I had last bumped into them back in July of 2011. That was the day I converted him from being a Cardinals fan into becoming a Braves fan. In fact, he was wearing the Braves hat I had given him that day at his check up this time around. It was well worn, which is a good thing, and I told him I had another hat just like it in my truck to replace the one he had. He said he would wear it, but that this hat was his "lucky hat" and he still wanted to wear it. I told him I fully understand, and that this hat could become his "even luckier" hat.

He was very receptive and said thanks. He has now grown into a seventh grader (Jr. High material). I asked how he was doing and he said he was playing baseball for his summer league team, doing well playing short stop and pitching, and that his leukemia still appeared to be in remission, although he was in Iowa City because he was more tired than usual. I told him that often happens when you are working hard at being a good ballplayer! His mom shared that they remember well the day we met in the pharmacy in 2009, and they always talk about the baseball tricks I showed him that day. I told Taylor and his mom I was very happy for them, and that I'm excited he is able to get back out and play! I shared what an impact he had on me that day in the pharmacy during my treatments by asking me when I could get back out and play again! He made me reset my goals to be able to get back out and play.

Taylor and his mom were getting ready to leave, so I walked them out of the Cancer Center and to their car. I took Taylor to my truck as I had an extra Braves hat behind the seat. (Always carry a spare!) I asked if he remembered the deal we had made back in 2011. He smiled and said, "You told me to keep playing and stay healthy so that when I turn fifteen, you can invite me to a Braves camp so you can watch me play." I then took the Braves cap out of my truck and put it on his head and said, "It's yours pal, and it can become your even luckier hat now."

Taylor is a great example of Regina's thought that it's all about "playing the hand you are dealt." Seeing his happy smile and having a chance to talk a little baseball was a good thing for both of us. I did share a thought with Taylor that I learned from Randy Pausch in his book *The Last Lecture,* "Be prepared. Luck is truly where preparation meets opportunity."

We talked about how hard work and preparation is important in both fighting cancer as well as working to be a good ball player. (A little luck along the way doesn't hurt either). Lots of parallels and lessons that can help each of us reach our individual dreams. I told him to never lose that determination, it's just too important, and it's truly what drives us.

We will both be looking forward to his fifteenth birthday and his chance to show me his "stuff" as we both work hard to pursue our individual dreams and to fight this disease. His grin was definitely the highlight of my summer! I truly believe Taylor and I both needed each other at just that moment, and God provided what I consider more than just a happenstance meeting between us.

An Encouraging Attitude

I told Taylor to never lose that determination,

It is just too important, and it's truly what drives us.

A Spiritual Insight

"Rejoice always, pray continually,
give thanks in all circumstances;
for this is God's will for you in Christ Jesus."
(1 Thessalonians 5:16-18)

A Step to Consider

"Be prepared. Luck is truly where preparation meets
opportunity."

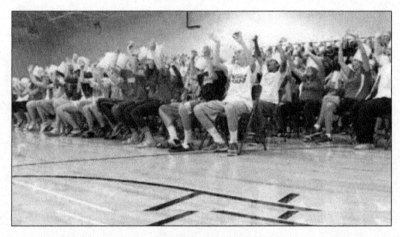

"Encouragement is a wonderful thing, and people do not receive enough during difficult times"

Reflection 31

Faith, Family, and Friends

October 7, 2013

One thing I've discovered over the past four years is not to desire the absence of problems in our lives. I have found it is actually pretty unrealistic since in this world we definitely will have troubles. We need to remember we have an eternity of problem free living reserved for us in heaven, which no one can take away.

As we face problems here on earth, we need to ask God's help to equip us to face them each day knowing that His hand never lets go of ours no matter what. Together, there is no challenge we can't handle. Along with God's hand, we can also find comfort and support from others who may be a part of our lives. I have had the joy of witnessing the supportive power of people I have been blessed to know, who have offered encouragement to me and to those I love.

A number of tests were run and I did receive some good news following the tests. I started the morning with labs, then chest X-ray. Labs show that my counts are now in the marginal range. That is much better than the counts back in July, which were in the abnormally high range. My chest X-ray was clear showing no cancer! My team of doctors feels the infection created the havoc and caused my counts to escalate. Given the fact we are still in the marginal zone, I will check back in three months and monitor any possible new symptoms closely. What a relief!

However, I received some sad news as my oncologist, Dr. "C" shared with me that he is retiring. His wife is going through her second bone marrow transplant and was having chemo today. He shared he needs to spend some quality time with her. He is quite a person and I am indebted to him for helping pull me through some very difficult times. I thanked him for all he has done for me as well as all those he has served at the University of Iowa Hospital Cancer Center.

He made sure he introduced me to my new doctor, whom he has worked with and trained. She is very pleasant and Dr. "C" said, "She follows the guidelines to a tee, just like me, so don't try to pull anything on her." He gave me a big grin, hand-shake, and hug, and left to be with his wife. Pretty emotional day for all!

"Often our prayers and faith don't save us from something, but rather they save us for something."

That statement has provided me a focus over the past four years. I often reflect on that as I've battled the anxieties and difficulties that go with living through cancer, and in turn, have firmly committed that I'm not about to give up! Having faith, family, and friends despite those uneasy and often painful times we face as cancer patients and survivors gives us the strength and stamina to continue.

I believe we can have an impact on others who may be facing similar trials and afflictions by modeling a positive and determined attitude as we battle this disease each and every day. Just could be that is what we are being saved for. As we struggle with whatever those afflictions may be in our lives, my hope is we will each take the opportunity to be open about those struggles and seek out faith and friends as a means of support as well as provide a measure of hope and comfort to others.

As has so often has happened, our students and staff came through with an incredible support project for one of our students who is battling leukemia and had just undergone a stem cell bone marrow transplant. The Holmes Art Department and a number of Holmes students showed their support for eighth grader, Will Reinart, by taking orders for yellow paper hats in recognition that September is Childhood Cancer Awareness Month. They then sold yellow paper hats at the beginning and end of the school day to help raise funds to support Will and his family during his treatments.

Students were given a yellow hat on Friday, September 27, during our Intervention/Enrichment period called, "Tiger Time." All the students and staff went to the gym and donned their hats to shoot a school wide video. The video will be shared with the Reinart family and the greater Holmes Junior High community via YouTube as a gesture of our caring support for Will and his family. The money raised along with the video was a way to show our school's support for the Reinart family. I have listed a link below to view the video as well as some links which share the story of our students and staff coming together to provide Will and his family the hope and comfort that only friends and family can provide during such a difficult time.

The Assembly helped me once again realize how important our friends and loved ones are when summoning the strength and courage to fight the battle against this disease. I feel so fortunate to have such a team in my dugout. Will and his family have all of us in their dugout pulling for him to rebuild and come back even stronger than ever, too! I am so proud of our students for rallying for Will and grateful for having them as a means of support to provide hope and comfort. There is no better place to have that happen than in our school and this community!

KWWL.com link on the "Yellow Hat" project:
http://www.kwwl.com/story/23555621/2013/09/28/cedar-falls-students-make-video-to-support-classmate-with-leukemia

"A Rally for Will": http://youtu.be/v5OELY6bo08

An Encouraging Attitude

I've discovered over the past four years not to desire the absence of problems in our lives.
It is pretty unrealistic since in this world we definitely will have troubles.

A Spiritual Insight

"I have told you these things, so that in me you may have peace.
In this world you will have trouble. But take heart!
I have overcome the world."
(Jesus in John 16:33)

A Step to Consider

You can have an impact on others who may be facing similar trials and afflictions
by modeling a positive and determined attitude in your own battle.

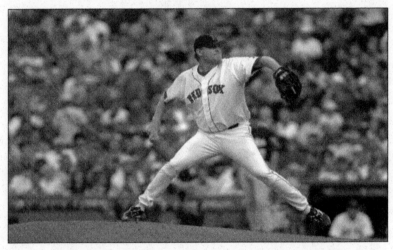

"Tough times don't last. Tough people do." - Curt Schilling

The Journey Continues...
2014

Reflection 32

Just Never Stop Hoping

February 23, 2014

I reached a special milestone, that being my fifth anniversary having been diagnosed with cancer. You may recall it was on my fifty-fifth birthday, five years ago, that I learned I had stage three-throat cancer and was not sure what the future would hold for me at that time. Well, here we are, five years later and I am fortunate enough to be celebrating my sixtieth birthday. I've been very fortunate to have the opportunity to feel the love and support of family, friends, students, and staff. There have certainly been some difficult times along the way, but also many reasons for joy and celebration.

I am of the belief that God doesn't save us from something, like the scourge of cancer, but rather saves us for something. I have had a number of friends and acquaintances over the past five years who have also battled cancer. Some are currently survivors like myself, and some have gone home, to never again have to feel the pain and suffering that cancer can bring not only to themselves, but also to those they love. I have shared many of the experiences I've had with people along the way. They have been so very meaningful to me. My next full checkup is scheduled for March 20 in Iowa City and I'm hopeful for good news as I cross that five-year anniversary threshold.

As you know, I have dealt with some of the ups and downs of my journey through reading and writing my reflections. I've often used baseball analogies to communicate those messages in an attempt to provide hope and comfort to those who may be facing similar journeys. Those of you who are baseball fans may be aware that another of my heroes, Curt Schilling, former hard-nosed pitcher for the Boston Red Sox, has recently been diagnosed with cancer. His wife Shonda is also a cancer survivor having been diagnosed back in 2001.

Curt's journey in the Major Leagues has been about toughness, one of the traits I have witnessed so many times from those who have battled this disease. That toughness has so often been demonstrated not only from a physical perspective, but also from a mental perspective. You may remember Curt from the 2004 American League Championship Series and the 2004 World Series. Curt displayed both physical and mental toughness in 2004 as he pitched in both series with a severe ankle tendon injury, and I'm confident will once again display the same toughness as he battles his cancer diagnosis. I've listed a brief summary of his 2004 pitching performance below:

> The Red Sox Organization stated on Oct. 13, 2004 that RHP Curt Schilling would need surgery on his right ankle whenever the season ended. At that time, it was unknown if Schilling would be able to pitch again during the postseason. But thanks to a breakthrough medical procedure, the Red Sox medical staff sutured the loose tendon on Schilling's right ankle, keeping it in place well enough for Schilling to be able to pitch effectively in Game 6 of the

American League Championship Series against the Yankees.

The sutures were removed after Game 6, and then re-inserted the day before he pitched Game 2 of the World Series against the Cardinals. With his tendon literally being held together by thread, Schilling allowed a total of one earned run over 13 innings in those final two starts of the postseason, both of which were wins.

As Curt says; "I've always believed life is about embracing the gifts and rising up to meet the challenges. We've been presented with another challenge, as I've recently been diagnosed with cancer. My father left me with a saying that I've carried my entire life and tried to pass on to our kids... Tough times don't last. Tough people do."

Couldn't think of a better approach to fighting cancer!

My reading has also brought me to a Blog site known as *"The Cure Baseball."* http://www.thecurebaseball.org/blog/

It's a site dedicated to using baseball to raise the hopes, spirits, and awareness for people and families affected by cancer. *"The Cure Baseball"* is a nonprofit organization that strives to positively impact the lives of people and families who have been affected by cancer through a collegiate summer baseball team. Its founder, Alex Paluka, lost his mother to breast cancer as a young boy and he has used the organization to tie baseball and cancer together in a unique and personal way. I was especially touched by a blog entry entitled HOPE. Yet another way baseball has been used to provide strength and comfort to those battling cancer.

HOPE.... by "The Cure Baseball"

When we see, read or hear the word hope we instinctively think of all that we hope and wish for in our own lives. When a person who is affected by cancer comes in contact with the word, they simply find strength. The word hope for these people echoes a message that there is light at the end of the tunnel that the battle they're fighting cannot take away their will to live and to beat cancer. Hope is a very strong word when you look at it. It provides no solid answers, no promises, but more or less a feeling that promotes the best and the battle in all of us. It's exactly what it means; hope is the feeling that no matter how unfavorable your odds may be, no matter how many doctors say you can't or won't make it, hope provides the will, the passion and the strength to continue to fight.

Hope has provided us with abilities that we may have never experienced without it. There have been days when we couldn't find the strength to get out of bed, a situation in our lives had taken away some of our strength, passion and lust for life. But it's always been hope and the possibility of a brighter future that has reinstated that strength, passion and lust for life in all of us. For people affected by cancer hope is sometimes all they have left to hang on to. The hope they'll see their kids one more time, hope the doctors will deliver good news or simply hope that they just stop hurting. Hope is not something we can buy, fake or fabricate. Hope knows no boundaries, ages, genders or races. It's free

*to everyone and always welcomes anyone who
wishes to embrace it.*

*Hope allows us to feel free, to feel strong and to
fight on. As tough a situation may be, hope finds
a way to ease the pain. What money cannot buy,
hope gladly provides. We see hope every day
we live, whether it's embedded in our own lives
or we become a witness to it. Hope is simple;
it's never far from grasp, although sometimes
it may seem like its miles away. Hope never
turns away in the toughest of times; it's always
waiting with open arms. Hope can be sparked
by anything, a color, a symbol or even a team.*

*Sometimes hope even seems to find us when we
least expect it, when we're at our worst, when
we can't even find the good in life. Hope lingers
with the ones who embrace it. Hope allows us
to hold on to it for as long as we want, it never
pushes us away, and many times hope opens
our eyes to the beauty of life. Hope can provide
the key to success, the water to our fountain of
youth and the strength to our battle.*

*So why do we lose hope? Do we get caught
up in numbers, figures, odds or even someone
else's opinions? Do we stray away from what
makes us smile, laugh and love? Do we simply
lose hope by losing our way, our mission or our
purpose? Hope never loses us, we always seem
to lose it. It is always the best feeling in the
world when we find hope again. But what if we
never lose it? What if we hope no matter what,
no matter how bleak the outcome looks or how*

backed into a corner we may feel? What if we hope for other people, what if our hope makes people find their own hope?

Just never stop HOPING!

The words toughness and hope bring to mind what I have witnessed from many of those I have been fortunate enough to meet and interact with during my five year journey with cancer. As we live out our lives embracing the gifts we have been given and rising up to meet the challenges we are faced with, remember, "Tough times don't last, but tough people do... if we keep hoping!"

An Encouraging Attitude

Hope can provide the key to success,
the water to our fountain of youth,
and the strength to our battle.
Just never stop HOPING!

A Spiritual Insight

Joshua said to them, "Do not be afraid; do not be discouraged.
Be strong and courageous.
This is what the LORD will do to all the enemies you are
going to fight."
(Joshua 10:25)

A Step to Consider

As we live out our lives embracing the gifts we have been given
and rising up to meet the challenges we are faced with,
remember,
"Tough times don't last, but tough people do... if we
keep hoping!"

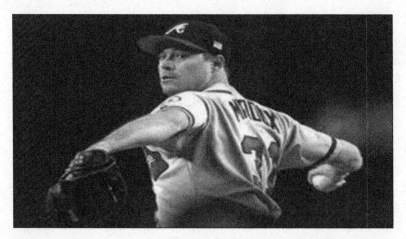

"Pitching is an art... It's about control, location and changing speeds."
- Greg Maddux

Reflection 33

The Art of Living

May 17, 2014

I have had several concerns arise following a recent hospitalization at Covenant in Waterloo. In short, the **Visiting Team** has **not** returned for extra innings, which is the good news. Tests in Iowa City confirmed that the cancer is still in remission. My doctors continue monitoring my lab counts as always to keep a close eye on things.

I've had some cardiac issues arise, which were the reason for my stay at Covenant. Lots of testing done and things are moving forward positively after making a few adjustments. Some genetics at play over which I have little control, but once again, I'm very thankful for my medical support both locally and in Iowa City.

I wanted to share some recent reading I have been doing as well. I seem to have had a bit more time while being laid up for a few days, so I picked up Max Lucado's, *"You'll Get Through This...Hope and Help for Turbulent Times."* You may know Max as he has also authored a number of inspirational Greeting Cards. His book is very good. I especially liked his chapter titled, *"Is God good when life isn't?"*

In the book, Max draws many parallels to turbulent times in our lives such as a traumatic injury or diagnosis, unemployment, a broken marriage, or divorce. He likens those times in our lives to the biblical story of Joseph being thrown in a pit.

> *"Joseph's pit came in the form of a cistern. Joseph was thrown into a hole and despised. Pits have no easy exit and Joseph's story got worse before it got better. Abandonment led to enslavement, entrapment, and imprisonment. He was sucker-punched. Sold out. Mistreated. People made promises only to break them. Offered gifts only to take them.*
>
> *As Max points out, "If hurt is a swampland, then Joseph was sentenced to a life of hard labor in the Everglades. Yet he never gave up. Bitterness never staked its claim. Anger never metastasized into hatred. His heart never hardened; resolve never vanished. He not only survived; he thrived. By the end of his life, Joseph was the second most powerful man of his generation. His life offers this lesson: in God's hands, intended evil becomes ultimate good. Joseph would be the first to tell you, life in the pit stinks. Yet, for all its rottenness, doesn't the pit do this much? It forces you to look upward. Someone from up there must come down here and give you a hand. God did for Joseph. And at the right time, in the right way, he will do the same for you."*

If there is one thing I've learned from my journey in life so far, it's that when we are faced with difficult times, we need to give control over to God. I've often struggled with this, as part of me wants to be in control at all times. It reminds me of something I heard one of my favorite players share at a pitching clinic one time. His name is Greg Maddux and he was one of the best control pitchers of all time. Of course, much of his success came during his time with the Atlanta Braves!

"Pitching is an art... it's not about blowing someone away with a 98 mph fastball... it's about control, location and changing speeds. I always threw hard enough, it took me a while to figure out how to throw slow enough..." - Greg Maddux

I draw an analogy to Greg's quote with how I'm hoping to adjust and live my life given some of the challenges that have been thrown my way. Living life is an art. So many times life's pace is so fast that we can get blown away as we race to keep up with the things that often get tossed our way in today's world. It can affect many things in our lives from our health, to our marriage, to our relationships with others. Life is about control, location, and changing speeds. Personally, I always have thrown hard in my life, and it has taken me a while to figure out how to throw slower. As for control, I have found by placing my troubles in God's hands and allowing Him to be in control, peace has entered where panic once resided and calmness settled in where anxiety once ruled. It's a comforting feeling.

The following quote sums up that strategy...

"This is the beginning of a new day. I can waste it or use it for good. What I do today is important because I am exchanging a day of my life for it. When tomorrow comes, this day will be gone forever, leaving in its place something I have traded for it. I want it to be a gain, not a loss; good, not evil; success, not failure--in order that I shall not regret the price I paid for it today." - Author unknown

This strategy helped me understand that I am exchanging each day of my life for the next 24 hours. I decided to spend my time by waking up each morning to live my day with intention.

I may not be able to choose my schedule and I certainly couldn't control the weather, the traffic, or whether there was bad news in my life. I could, however, decide how I would react to all those things that ultimately would determine whether I enjoyed my day or not. I needed to slow down and live each day with intention!

An Encouraging Attitude

Art of Living
By Max Lucado
You'll get through this.
It won't be painless.
It won't be quick.
But God will use this mess for good.
Don't be foolish or naïve.
But don't despair either.
With God's help, you'll get through this.

A Spiritual Insight

"This is the day the Lord has made;
let us rejoice and be glad in it."
(Psalm 118:24)

A Step to Consider

Place your troubles in God's hands and allow Him to be in control.
When you do, peace will enter where panic once resided and calmness will settle in where anxiety once ruled.

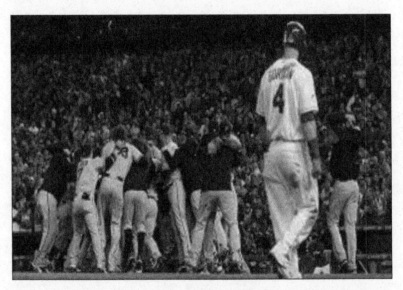

Overcoming Adversity With The "No Complaining Rule"

Reflection 34

Pick Up the Pace

October 26, 2014

I had a recent visit to Iowa City given some ongoing concerns with the side effects of treatments, and the good news is that my counts have once again returned to the normal range and I'm working through those ongoing side effects.

As I shared in my last Reflection, I had some cardiac issues, which were corrected with the implant of a pacemaker in July and I was just recently cleared of restrictions that had been put in place at the time of the implant. Darned genetics at play of which I have little control, but once again, I'm very thankful for the medical support I have received and the fact the pacemaker has allowed me to once again "pick up the pace"! Which is something often needed here as principal at the Junior High.

It was October, a time when baseball playoffs and the World Series always get my adrenaline going. A quote I read which has been credited to Theo Epstein, of the Chicago Cubs gave me some pause, as his words not only applied to the team sport of baseball, but they also applied to the team sport of life.

> "Human beings can accomplish more when they are doing it for others, rather than just for themselves." - Theo Epstein

As I thought about it, these words actually applied to both the San Francisco Giants and the Kansas City Royals who played their way into the 2014 World Series. Both teams were playing for their cities, families, and had an extremely loyal fan base that spanned generations. But perhaps most importantly, both teams were full of players who were playing for each member of their respective teams.

In post-game interviews throughout the World Series, players being interviewed talked about the love they had for their fellow players, their brothers. They talked about having each other's back, when one player was struggling, the others stepped up. The word "I" was rarely used, "we" was the preferred word. All the players were playing for each other by doing the very best that they could in whatever role they individually played.

As a team, the Giants achieved a well-deserved World Series championship. As a team, the Kansas City Royals, riddled with injuries the entire playoffs, exceeded everyone's expectations, except perhaps their own. Despite the challenges both teams faced, there was no complaining along the way. What a great lesson in life, learning to lean on others in challenging times while not complaining about, but rather overcoming hardships along the way! It was and is what my **Home Team** has been all about!

Just as the Royals and Giants have found ways to overcome adversity to get to the Fall Classic without complaining, we too can face challenges with the help of those around us.

This year's World Series teams (Giants and Royals) have done a good job of taking some of the negatives that have happened during their regular seasons, and without complaining, have come up with some innovative solutions to get their teams to the October classic. Whether its Giants catcher Buster Posey returning to MVP form after a season ending leg injury in 2011, or the Royals hot hitting first baseman Eric Hosmer coming back from a serious August hand injury, they have both found ways to be positive contributors.

I've taken a note or two on their teams "no complaining rules" and have tried to apply them to my life. As I've watched others I care for suffer and battle cancer and all the nasty things it brings with it, it would be easy to fall into the trap of complaining. I wanted to share some recent reading I have been doing about complaining as I find it helpful to try to fill my mind with positive thoughts and avoid that trap that can be so easy to fall into.

Two books, *The No Complaining Rule,* by Jon Gordon and *A Complaint Free World,* by Will Bowen have provided some positive thoughts that I have taken with me on a daily basis. Those thoughts help me to look at ways to turn potential negatives into positives, while realizing that any constructive changes we make in the world must first start with ourselves. Jon Gordon sums up those thoughts in a brief reflection with some of his writing below.

Life and Death by Jon Gordon

Two weeks ago my family and I were on a plane from LAX heading to Atlanta. Shortly after taking off and soaring above 10,000 feet the plane abruptly slowed down and the power went out as the pilot spoke over the sound system, "We're experiencing a mechanical failure and heading back for an emergency landing."

The next moment the plane descended so rapidly that my head hurt and I thought we were going down. I looked at my wife and son, who were sitting to the left and a few rows back since we couldn't get seats together, and saw the fear in my wife's eyes. I grabbed my daughter's hand as she sat in the seat directly in front of me.

She asked, "Should I be scared Dad?"

"Just pray," I said.

This can't be happening, I thought. We're not ready to die. I still have three more books that I know I'm meant to write. I grabbed my phone and tweeted that we were making an emergency landing at LAX and if we didn't make it that I love everyone. A few minutes later the plane leveled off as I watched off duty airline employees, who were sitting in passenger seats, get up and run to the back of the plane. The pilot announced that we were going to make an emergency landing and to brace for impact. He said there would be emergency vehicles there to meet us and that the flight attendants were trained on what to do when we landed.

While everything seemed eerily calm and quiet I couldn't stop thinking about the plane catching on fire or splitting in two when we landed.

Miraculously and thankfully we made a safe landing. The pilot said there was a fire in one of the engines but when we landed the fire was extinguished.

When we walked off the plane my 14-year-old son put his arm around me and said, "It means we have more work to do Dad. God has a plan for us."

What a good way to look at life, especially after facing the possible loss of it, something all cancer patients experience when diagnosed. We all are faced with many challenges in life, and it can be so easy to fall into a complaining mode when those challenges come knocking on our door. Just as the Royals and Giants have found ways to overcome adversity to get to the Fall Classic without complaining, we too can face challenges with the help of those around us, what I would refer to as my **Home Team**.

Instead of complaining when hardships come our way, lean on those **Home Team** members and show your gratitude for their help. As inspirational writer, William Arthur Ward writes, "Feeling gratitude and not expressing it is like wrapping a present and not giving it." Let's remember that it is not enough to be grateful for the people and things of your life. For your gratitude to impact others you must also express it. After all, we **all** have more work to do according to God's plan!

An Encouraging Attitude

We **all** have more work to do according to God's plan!

A Spiritual Insight

"Do everything without grumbling or arguing,
so that you may become blameless and pure,
children of God without fault in a warped and
crooked generation.
Then you will shine among them like stars in the sky."
(Apostle Paul while in a Roman prison - Philippians 2:14-15)

A Step to Consider

Instead of complaining when hardships come our way,
lean on those **Home Team** members and show your gratitude
for their help.

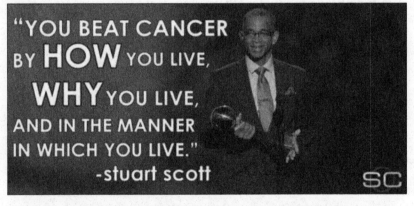

"You beat cancer by how you live, why you live, and in the manner in which you live." - Stuart Scott, ESPN Anchor

The Journey Continues...
2015

Reflection 35

Life's Warnings

January 7, 2015

As the cold winter months set in, my schedule had returned to its typically busy pace. I hadn't really slowed down much since I'd had the pacemaker procedure, and my energy and stamina levels began to take a hit. It has always been hard for me to slow down, even after the cancer treatment regimen had totally drained me. I felt as though I had to squeeze the most out of every day, not knowing how and when the days might end.

I needed to find some balance, and I discovered some wonderful balancing thoughts in Jon Gordon's book, *The Carpenter*. In addition, one of my favorite sports broadcasters, Stuart Scott fell victim to cancer. Jon's book taught me the importance of slowing down and Stuart's legacy taught me about living with rather than battling cancer. Once again, I believe God provided me the wisdom to continue my journey by bringing Jon and Stuart's experiences into my life.

The Carpenter is filled with many powerful lessons. It's about a young man named Michael who wakes up in the hospital with a bandage on his head and fear in his heart. The stresses of building a growing business with his wife Sarah caused him to collapse while on a morning jog. When Michael finds out the man who saved his life is a Carpenter, he visits him and quickly learns that he is more than just a Carpenter; he is also a builder of lives, careers, people, and teams.

As the Carpenter shares his wisdom, Michael attempts to save his business in the face of adversity, rejection, fear, and failure. Along the way, he learns that there's no such thing as an overnight success, but that there are timeless principles to help you make an impact on people and the world around you. One of those lessons included, **"Remember, life gives us warnings for a reason. Learn from this. Do things differently."**

As I have come to realize and others have shared, sometimes the pace at which we are expected to perform in today's world can divert us from what really matters. The fact is we should slow down, taking time to love life, and enjoy all of it while fearing none of it. Certainly, that thought is great advice, but my experience is that it's not always easy to live out. Another relevant lesson the Carpenter shared included:

"When you love, you serve, and when you serve, you sacrifice. Service requires a sacrifice of something. Whether it's time, energy, money, love, effort, or focus, serving others always costs you something, but with service and sacrifice, you gain so much more."

Life truly is about loving, caring for, and serving others, along with the joy it can bring in our lives each and every day.

As many of you may also know, the sports industry also lost a great individual, as Stuart Scott, a longtime anchor at ESPN, died at the age of forty-nine. As I've shared in past reflections, most of us have been touched by cancer in some way, shape or form. It has always bothered me that we often refer to people who have died as a result of cancer as having "lost their fight with cancer." I recall watching Stuart during his ESPY speech earlier in 2014, and I thought his remarks about not losing the fight when you die, but instead winning the fight in how you live were truly inspirational.

As I watched the tributes, read the articles, followed the tweets and posts following Stuart's death, the words that people used to describe him touched me. Passionate, energetic, courageous, fighter, dynamic, fearless, game-changer, dad, friend, and leader were some of those words used to describe Stuart and his life.

Those words certainly described what I think Stuart stood for in his life, both when he was healthy, as well as after he was diagnosed and was fighting this disease. How he lived, why he lived, and the manner in which he lived are a true testament to the quote he used when he received the "Jimmy V" Perseverance Award in 2014, "You beat cancer by how you live, why you live, and in the manner in which you live."

You can view Stuart's full speech at this link if interested: https://www.youtube.com/watch?v=Yl_0ieqSi7Q

That speech inspired me to think about the manner in which we live each and every day. Make the most of every day. Enjoy the people around you. Inspire others with your actions, your attitude, your words, and your effort. If you get knocked down, pick yourself up. If someone else gets knocked down, help pick him or her up. Obviously, that's not always easy to do, and I'll be the first to admit I've not always been successful at that. It's certainly something to strive for, and Stuart's example helps me work toward that goal each day.

As a good friend recently shared, "A New Year is a reset button. Let's control what we can control—which starts with our attitude, our energy, and our work ethic—and it will lead to amazing things in 2015."

If you haven't had a chance to watch this tribute to Stuart Scott, I encourage you to take the time and view it at this link. http://espn.go.com/video/clip?id=espn:12118361

An Encouraging Attitude

"Remember, life gives us warnings for a reason.
Learn from this. Do things differently."
— Jon Gordon from his book, *"The Carpenter."*

A Spiritual Insight

"I know what it is to be in need, and I know
what it is to have plenty.
I have learned the secret of being content in any
and every situation,
whether well fed or hungry, whether living
in plenty or in want."
(Apostle Paul reflecting on his life of service to God in
Philippians 4:12)

A Step to Consider

Make the most of every day. Enjoy the people around you.
Inspire others with your actions, your attitude, your words,
and your effort.
If you get knocked down, pick yourself up.
If someone else gets knocked down, help pick him or her up.

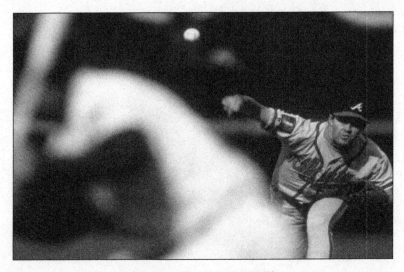

Fix Your Eyes on the Ball!

Reflection 36

Onward

May 16, 2015

The spring months included a number of difficult days. I needed to clear my mind and find a focus, but more importantly, I needed a dose of calm! Those difficult days reminded me that the world is full of trouble and afflictions and we certainly get plenty of those reminders on the daily news each day. Even though hardships are part of our life's journey, we can overcome them by looking to God. He is meting hardships out to us while at the same time training us to overcome them, unfettered by our circumstances.

I tried hard not to dwell on what had gone wrong along the way, but rather focus on what to do next, spending my time and energy moving forward to find solutions to the challenges. I once again recalled he time I requested a phone repair ticket on our home landline when a message popped up to move to the next option saying, "ONWARD."

We shouldn't get stuck in what just happened, but instead let it go and keep moving "onward" to help comfort those who suffered the loss, "onward" to the next treatment, and "onward" to the next at-bat or next pitch. It sounds simple, but think about how many times a day something negative happens. By quickly regrouping and letting those things go, we can move "onward."

As we all face a number of issues each and every day that seem to demand our attention, I wanted to focus on what has helped me get through some difficult days in the past month. The month has included thoughts on dealing with the pace that life tends to throw our way on a regular basis. "Pesky" side effects from cancer treatments, as well as the heartache that comes our way with the passing of those who may be close to us have also been a part of the past month. Recently, life has been a blur for me and it has been hard to keep a balance and focus on the things that need my attention.

My mind raced with thoughts on how to deal with these issues and caused some restlessness over the past month. I kept coming back to some advice my college baseball coach; John Paulsen gave me about focus.

"To be successful, you have to fix your eyes and focus on the ball, blocking out all those things that may be whirling around in your mind competing for your focus and attention."

My dad had been battling Parkinson's the past few years and it was difficult to see him fight the disease with the grit and determination he had modeled his whole life for me. He developed pneumonia on April 24, and went home to be with his loving Father on Sunday, April 26. As I dealt with all those issues that go through a person's mind when faced with losing a loved one, I read from Sarah Young's *Jesus Calling* devotional Friday morning, and it immediately brought me peace.

"MAKE ME YOUR FOCAL POINT as you move through this day. Just as a spinning ballerina must keep her eyes on a given point to main- tain her balance, so you must keep returning your focus to Me. Circumstances are in flux, and the world seems to be whirling around you. The only way to keep your balance is to fix your

*eyes on Me, the One who never changes. If
you gaze too long at your circumstances, you
will become dizzy and confused. Look to me,
refreshing yourself in My Presence, and your
steps will be steady and sure (Hebrews 12:2;
Psalm 102:27)."*

Just as my coach had shared that to be successful on the
diamond, you have to fix your eyes and focus on the ball, I
once again realized that the "ball" in our daily lives is Jesus,
and that our focus needs to be on Him each and every day. He
will refresh us daily and help keep us on balance when we so
often get dizzy and confused with the whirlwind of things that
come our way.

Dad taught me many things as I grew up. At times, he had
what some would consider a tough exterior, but we always
knew there was a large, warm, and caring heart inside. (Just
didn't want to mess up to see that exterior side of him!) He
often had a sense of humor when dealing with difficult situations, yet faced them head on without complaining. He rarely
talked about his service to our Country until his later years, just
as so many of his generation did. He taught us all to be fighters,
to work hard, and to stick up for what we believe is right. His
final hours demonstrated that, and his spirit for life and living
will live on with us all forever.

Robert Welter's Obituary:
http://wcfcourier.com/lifestyles/announcements/obitu-
aries/robert-m-welter/article_e81705fa-396c-521e-8e56-
f3b8b73429e0.html

A good friend shared a verse that was especially comforting
as we spent our final hours together with dad as a family.

God saw you getting tired and a cure was
not to be.
So he put His arms around you and whispered,
"Come to Me."[8]

Those words truly brought comfort to me, and I'm sure they will as well to those who are facing diseases such as Parkinson's and cancer. May we each get focused on what is truly important each day, blocking out all those things that may be whirling around in our minds and are competing for our focus and attention. As we encounter problems that seem to have no immediate solution, our responses can either take us up or down. We can lash out at the difficulty, resenting it and feeling sorry for ourselves which will take us down into a pit of self-pity. Or we can use it as a chance to see it from a higher perspective, being that the obstacle frustrating you is only a light and momentary trouble. Once our perspective is heightened, our focus can be taken away from the problem altogether and placed back on Jesus to be refreshed in His daily presence.

An Encouraging Attitude

My coach said, "You have to fix your eyes and
focus on the ball."
I once again realized that the "ball" in our daily lives is Jesus,
and that our focus needs to be on Him each and every day.

A Spiritual Insight

"Therefore, since we are surrounded by such a
great cloud of witnesses,
let us throw off everything that hinders and the sin
that so easily entangles.

---

[8] From: God Saw You Getting Tired, by Frances and Kathleen Coelho

And let us run with perseverance the race marked out for us."
(Hebrews 12:1)

A Step to Consider

Focus away from the problem altogether
and place it back on Jesus to be refreshed in His
daily presence.

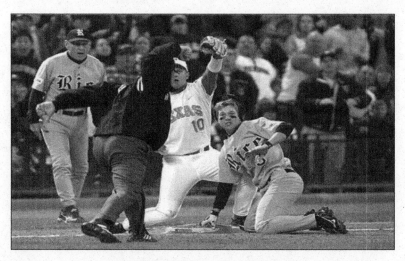

Setbacks Life May Toss Our Way

Reflection 37

Setbacks

October 10, 2015

I just had my regular checkup in Iowa City this past week and things are looking positive with regard to my counts. I've developed a routine of sorts to deal with the side effects of treatments. There are ups and downs, but I'm happy to report, mostly ups! I again want to offer a special thanks to my doctors and medical support team for the time and efforts they have given to assist me. Unfortunately, I have discovered thanks is often a forgotten word in today's society.

A number of thoughts entered my mind when faced with the tests and challenges I've experienced over the past six years. Whether those challenges were health related, work related or relationship related, as soon as my mind got snagged on a problem, I did my best to take it to God. Often easier said than done, but one thing I've found is that when I turn my thoughts to God, the problem seems to fade in significance.

Often I find myself not thinking about what is confronting me today, but what may be

happening in the future. However, it gives me peace to lift that problem out of my mind and deposit it into the future knowing that together, with God's help and guidance we will handle it. Seems to help release me from my negative thoughts so I can deal with today.

As I watched the Cubs battle the Pirates in the NLCS this fall, I couldn't help but notice that there is an upside to setbacks. Both teams faced many struggles over the year, but they overcame them to reach the playoffs. I drew many comparisons to the obstacles I have faced and took note of how both teams handled the adversities that came their way. Setbacks can help plant the seeds for new dreams in each of our lives and provide great life lessons for each of us. Those struggles we battle can help motivate us to reach new heights in our lives if we will let them.

I have to admit, it's not always easy to adopt this mindset when faced with the "curveballs" life tosses our way, but by adopting it, we can deepen our relationships with others and most importantly, with God. They also provide the opening to learn some lessons that success cannot teach by developing in us the kind of patience that waits on God, and in turn, trusts Him for the strength to endure.

I have several close friends and colleagues who are experiencing difficult trials and setbacks at this time with family and friends. I know they are being tested just as I know many of us are being tested. My prayers are extended their way, knowing that God will provide the patience and strength to endure those trials.

Just as Pirate and Cub fans were reaching out, hoping that the battle they faced against each other in the one game playoff would go their way, we need to remember that both clubs had overcome setbacks along the way to reach the goal of being a playoff contender. Both clubs endured and persevered! Anyone who works to overcome the challenges of life's struggles needs to take on a "survivor's mindset" by enduring and persevering.

For those of you who are Cub fans, congratulations on your 4-0 win and may the success continue. For those of you who are Pirate fans, congratulations on a great season! For both clubs, and for each of us, please remember a thought that was shared with me recently by a great friend.

"The man who is at the peak and the one who just failed are exactly in the same position. Each must decide what they will do next." - Jigoro Kano

An Encouraging Attitude

Setbacks can help plant the seeds for new dreams
in each of our lives
and provide great life lessons for each of us.

A Spiritual Insight

"Consider it pure joy my brothers and sisters,
whenever you face trials of many kinds,
because you know that the testing of your
faith produces perseverance."
(James 1:2-3)

A Step to Consider

May we each decide to endure and persevere
to reach new heights in our lives despite what trials
and setbacks life may toss our way!

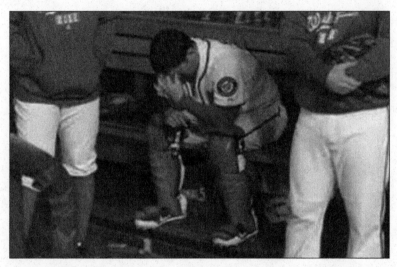

"Don't let yesterday take up too much of today" - Will Rogers

The Journey Continues...
2016

Reflection 38
Shut the Door on Yesterday

January 2, 2016

O n some days, it seemed I was able to cope with my physical hardships, while on other days, I just wanted out. One thing was for certain, God was always there to help me on those "other" days! I learned perseverance through enduring a wide range of challenges and I think that nicely sums up my life's journey to this point.

Life can be messy in the sense that things don't always go exactly according to our plans. Our kids may have problems, our health may not be what we would like it to be, our careers don't always go as we'd like, and we can generally count on the fact that we are going to make some mistakes along the way.

That's okay because we need to embrace it. It is what makes us real. It's what makes us human. It is all part of the story of our lives that we add a new chapter to each day. The struggles that we've had can certainly help teach others. The fact that we've kept going despite obstacles, setbacks, and mistakes can help motivate and inspire others.

As we add those new chapters, I've discovered that we can't let yesterday take up too much of today. The following reflection shares my experiences with a couple I met in Iowa City during a follow up medical visit as well as some advice I received long ago from one of my coaches. Both of these experiences offered some genuine, real life learning.

As I was sitting in Iowa City this past week waiting for one of my appointments, I had the opportunity to sit and visit with an elderly couple in the waiting room that were dealing with some significant pain issues following their treatments. We got into a discussion regarding what some of the remedies were that they had been investigating to help relieve the pain, and we compared notes. Both were extremely upbeat and happy despite their pain issues. One of the thoughts they shared really landed home for me.

"Despite our physical issues, we have each other and we don't let yesterday take up much of today."

That struck home with me as it brought back a thought that was drilled into my head during my playing days, which I shared often with my own players when coaching. I think my coach borrowed the thought from Will Rogers, but it has served me well throughout the years.

**"Don't let yesterday take up too much of today." –
Will Rogers**

That thought represents the approach I have always tried to take as a teacher, coach, administrator, and yes, **especially as a cancer survivor.** We need to be reminded of this constantly as it's so easy to fall into the trap of self-pity as we struggle with physical, emotional, and spiritual issues that often confront us as survivors on a daily basis.

I recall in my playing days when I may have struggled at the plate hitting on a given day, I couldn't let my mind drift as I needed to continue to focus on the rest of my game for the team to have a chance at being successful. Lesson learned— Don't live in the past, you can't do anything about the past. It will never change whether it's yesterday or last year. The future is yet to be determined and can be influenced by what you do today. Today is the only day that really matters. That lesson is one that has served me well on a daily basis!

Vivian Laramore Rader, Florida's "forgotten poet" writes:

> I have shut the door on yesterday,
> its sorrows and mistakes.
> I have locked within its gloomy walls
> past failures and mistakes.
> And now I throw the key away,
> and seek another room.
> And furnish it with hope and smiles,
> and every spring-time bloom.
> No thought shall enter this abode
> that has a taint of pain.
> And envy, malice, and distrust
> shall never entrance gain.
> I have shut the door on yesterday
> and thrown the key away.
> Tomorrow holds no fear for me,
> since I have found today.

I have found this poem inspirational as I move forward each day. I am joyful that I have the opportunity to continue to experience the simple joys that life brings. Joys such as hugging my grandchildren, Grace and Lucy, as well as enjoying the life experiences of my children as they move forward in their own lives. Despite some of the physical, emotional, and spiritual pains that life can bring our way, these are things that must be cherished and will help us pull together and be supported as we move forward. The elderly couple in the waiting room was right, despite our physical issues, we all have each other and we shouldn't let yesterday take up much of today.

As I've often shared, I enjoy reading to help process my thoughts about moving forward. I have especially enjoyed John Burke's new book titled, *Imagine Heaven*. For decades, Burke has been studying accounts of survivors brought back from near death who lived to tell of both heavenly and hellish experiences. Burke shows how the common experiences shared by thousands of survivors —including doctors, college professors, bank presidents, people of all ages and cultures, and even blind people —point to the exhilarating picture of Heaven promised us in the Bible. It has helped me gain an inspiring view of the life to come and ways we can live our lives today so that we don't let yesterday take up too much of today. You may even discover, as I have, that Heaven is even more amazing than you've ever imagined!

An Encouraging Attitude

"We can't let yesterday take up too much of today." – Will Rogers

A Spiritual Insight

"Forget the former things; do not dwell on the past." (God to His people in Isaiah 43:18)

A Step to Consider

Take every opportunity to continue to experience the simple
joys that life brings.
Joys such as hugging your spouse, children, and
grandchildren.

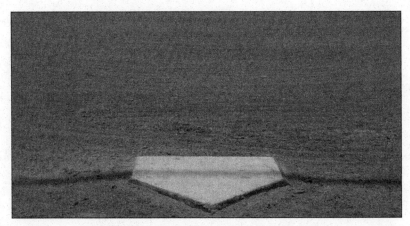

Don't Widen Home Plate - Coach John Scolinos

Reflection 39

Accountability

April 2, 2016

Throughout my treatment regimen, I constantly heard patients talking about quick and easy solutions to help alleviate their medical problems. Often, they didn't care much about what the solution involved, as long as their problem got resolved quickly and easily. What they didn't realize were the hidden dangers that often accompanied taking short cuts.

I discovered I couldn't allow the temptation of quick short-cuts to my personal wellness fool me. As in most everything, there are no easy short cuts to achieving our goals, whether those goals involve our health, our careers or even our families.

The following reflection shares some thoughts and experiences regarding taking shortcuts, not only on the playing field, but also outside of the playing field. These are lessons that have impacted me, whether with family, friends, teams, my career, and yes, even in dealing with cancer.

I've had a few bumps in the road the past few weeks leading to a visit to Iowa City. The good news is it appears my hearing loss following treatments has begun to stabilize. That's certainly a relief! I have some interesting technology in place to deal with that issue. Things have been up and down with my counts, and I am awaiting some lab results. I continue my daily routines to deal with the side effects of treatments. As we near the end of another school year, I have much to be grateful for.

As I was sitting in Iowa City this past week waiting for my appointment, once again I had the opportunity to sit and visit with a couple in the waiting room as they waited with their teenage children at the Pharmacy. One of the children had been recently diagnosed with cancer and they were struggling as they waited to pick up a prescription for him. We got into a discussion about the improvements made in treating cancer, and the improved success rate with surviving the disease. They wanted to hear about my experience, so I shared a brief summary, doing my best to share the positive outcome, and I think they appreciated that.

One thing led to another and the discussion turned to raising a young family these days and all the challenges that it involves. We agreed that times have changed over the years, and that often, there seems to be a lack of constants in place these days with young people similar to when they were growing up. That struck home with me being in the "education business" as I deal with young people and their parents every day.

That brought to mind a presentation that was shared with me back in my early coaching days by Coach John Scolinos, who coached baseball a very long time at Cal Poly, Pomona. Coach was presenting at an ABCA Coaches National Convention back in the mid '90s, and it reminded me of a message that I often shared with my players. Thoughts that had an impact outside of the playing field and that could be carried with us in each of our life's journeys, whether it be with family, friends, teams, careers or dealing with cancer.

Posted in: Coaching, Family Values and Youth baseball blog

by John O'Sullivan:

In 1996, Coach Scolinos was 78 years old and five years retired from a college coaching career that began in 1948. He shuffled to the stage at the ABCA Convention in Nashville to an impressive standing ovation, wearing dark polyester pants, a light blue shirt, and a string around his neck from which home plate hung — a full-sized, stark-white home plate.

After speaking for twenty-five minutes, not once mentioning the prop hanging around his neck, Coach Scolinos appeared to notice the snickering among some of the coaches. Even those who knew Coach Scolinos had to wonder exactly where he was going with this, or if he had simply forgotten about home plate since he'd gotten on stage. Then, finally ...

"You're probably all wondering why I'm wearing home plate around my neck. Or maybe you think I escaped from Camarillo State Hospital," he said, his voice growing irascible. I laughed along with the others, acknowledging the possibility. "No," he continued, "I may be old, but I'm not crazy. The reason I stand before you today is to share with you baseball people what I've learned in my life, what I've learned about home plate in my 78 years. "Several hands went up when Scolinos asked how many Little League coaches were in the room. "Do you know how wide home plate is in Little League?" After a pause, someone offered,

217

"Seventeen inches," more question than answer. "That's right," he said. "How about in Babe Ruth? Any Babe Ruth coaches in the house?" Another long pause. "Seventeen inches?" came a guess from another reluctant coach. "That's right," said Scolinos. "Now, how many high school coaches do we have in the room?" Hundreds of hands shot up, as the pattern began to appear. "How wide is home plate in high school baseball?" "Seventeen inches," they said, sounding more confident. "You're right!" Scolinos barked. "And you college coaches, how wide is home plate in college?" "Seventeen inches!" we said, in unison. "Any Minor League coaches here? How wide is home plate in pro ball?" "Seventeen inches!" "RIGHT! And in the Major Leagues, how wide home plate is in the Major Leagues?" "Seventeen inches!"

"SEV-EN-TEEN INCHES!" he confirmed, his voice bellowing off the walls. "And what do they do with a Big League pitcher who can't throw the ball over seventeen inches?" Pause. "They send him to Pocatello!" he hollered, drawing raucous laughter.

"What they don't do is this: they don't say, 'Ah, that's okay, Jimmy. You can't hit a seventeen-inch target? We'll make it eighteen inches, or nineteen inches. We'll make it twenty inches so you have a better chance of hitting it. If you can't hit that, let us know so we can make it wider still, say twenty-five inches.'"

Pause.
"Coaches ..."
Pause.

" ... What do we do when our best player shows up late to practice? When our team rules forbid facial hair and a guy shows up unshaven? What if he gets caught drinking? Do we hold him accountable? Or do we change the rules to fit him, do we widen home plate?

The chuckles gradually faded, as four thousand coaches grew quiet, the fog lifting as the old coach's message began to unfold. He turned the plate toward himself and, using a Sharpie, began to draw something. When he turned it toward the crowd, point up, a house was revealed, complete with a freshly drawn door and two windows. "This is the problem in our homes today. With our marriages, with the way we parent our kids. With our discipline. We don't teach accountability to our kids, and there is no consequence for failing to meet standards. We widen the plate!"

Pause.

Then, to the point at the top of the house he added a small American flag. "This is the problem in our schools today. The quality of our education is going downhill fast and teachers have been stripped of the tools they need to be successful, and to educate and discipline our young people. We are allowing others to widen home plate! Where is that getting us?"

Silence...

He replaced the flag with a Cross. "And this is the problem in the Church, where powerful people in positions of authority have taken advantage of young children, only to have such an atrocity swept under the rug for years. Our church leaders are widening home plate!"

I was amazed. At a baseball convention where I expected to learn something about curveballs and bunting and how to run better practices, I had learned something far more valuable. From an old man with home plate strung around his neck, I had learned something about life, about myself, about my own weaknesses and about my responsibilities as a leader. I had to hold myself and others accountable to that which I knew to be right, lest our families, our faith, and our society continue down an undesirable path.

"If I am lucky," Coach Scolinos concluded, "you will remember one thing from this old coach today. It is this: if we fail to hold ourselves to a higher standard, a standard of what we know to be right; if we fail to hold our spouses and our children to the same standards, if we are unwilling or unable to provide a consequence when they do not meet the standard; and if our schools and churches and our government fail to hold themselves accountable to those they serve, there is but one thing to look forward to ..."

With that, he held home plate in front of his chest, turned it around, and revealed its dark black backside. "... dark days ahead."

Coach Scolinos died in 2009 at the age of 91, but not before touching the lives of hundreds of players and coaches, including mine. Meeting him at my first ABCA convention kept me returning year after year, looking for similar wisdom and inspiration from other coaches. He is the best clinic speaker the ABCA has ever known, because he was so much more than a baseball coach.

Coach's message was relevant in 1996, and it still is today. His message was clear:

"Coaches, keep your player—no matter how good they are—your own children, and most of all, keep yourself at seventeen inches, DON'T WIDEN THE PLATE."

I can clearly recall sitting in my chemo and radiation treatments in Iowa City, having a frank discussion with my oncologist, Dr. "C" as I struggled with the nausea from chemo and the pain in my throat from radiation. I asked Dr. "C" if I could cut the treatments short as they appeared to be working and shrinking the tumors in my neck, and his reply was simply, "Dave, I feel terrible I have to put you through this, but in the end it will all work out for you."

He was compassionate, but he didn't "widen the plate." Yes, it did work out successfully for me thanks to Dr. "C" holding me to what he knew was right by having me follow the precise treatment regimen he had prescribed with no short cuts!

An Encouraging Attitude

I discovered I couldn't allow the temptation of quick shortcuts fool me as I moved forward toward my personal wellness goal.

A Spiritual Insight

"But thanks be to God! He gives us the victory through our
Lord Jesus Christ.
Therefore, my dear brothers and sisters, stand firm. Let
nothing move you."
(1 Corinthians 15:57-58)

A Step to Consider

Let's work together to hold ourselves and our families to a
similar standard
of what we know to be right each and every day,
by not taking short cuts and widening the plate
as we face the trials and challenges put before us each and
every day.

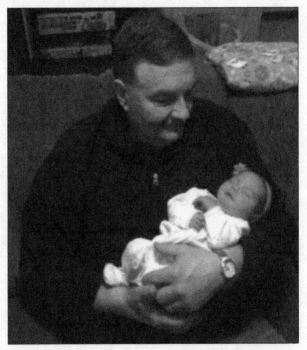

"Grandpa never gave in, and he never gave up."

Reflection 40

All for Naught?

April 16, 2016

The following reflection was the most difficult for me to write. I had wrestled with the idea of retirement for a number of years, while battling the ongoing challenges that cancer had brought into my life. I felt, as I had mentioned in an earlier reflection, that God may have saved me for something, and that something was to continue working with kids.

My heart and soul have always been in serving others, especially kids, so it was a natural battle trying to make the decision. I have always been surrounded by love when making difficult decisions and this situation was no different. Each day, I watched the students and thought not only of the impact I could have on them going forward, but also the impact they so often had on me.

My mind was once again in "analyzer mode" and after weighing all the factors and praying on it long and hard, I decided it was time to make a decision. The questions most often asked of me when working with my students centered on whether or not I cared about them, their future, their life, and their wellbeing. I could honestly say yes when answering those questions, and felt it was now time to move forward and take that same passion to other things in my life while I still had the energy and health to do so.

The secret to life and the greatest success strategy of all is, "Love all of it and fear none of it!" – Jon Gordon

Many teammates during my baseball playing days said to me after their retirement from the game, "Dave, ride it till the wheels fall off because once it's over it's over." Well, my wheels may not be completely off, but there are a lot of miles on these old tires, and the treads left on them are a bit thinner. My body just doesn't want to do what it used to do and I've always said that if I couldn't perform to the level I'm accustomed to, then it was time to walk away.

Baseball and life are games of failure that tend to always be followed by opportunity, if given the chance. Baseball is also a game that can provide many lessons that can be applied to life. It teaches life lessons that I don't think any other profession could teach and from which I have drawn many parallels in my years in education. Baseball (as life) is also about the journey we each travel, not necessarily our ultimate destination. We all have something to learn from the game by pushing aside the fear of failure that can come from taking on challenges to grow on our journey.

As the old adage says, "All good things must come to an end," so after forty years in education as a teacher, coach, athletic director, and principal, I have made the decision to hang up my cleats and retire as Holmes Jr. High's Principal at the end of this contract season. I have been **blessed** beyond measure. My cup has been filled with many good times and much good fortune. I have chased a lot of dreams for the past forty years, allowing me to meet some of the most amazing characters you could ever imagine, while also allowing me to experience lasting relationships that most people could only dream of.

I can honestly say that I worked hard, prepared, and always did my best to serve my students and staff to the best of my ability. I have great respect for the education profession and those in it, and have always tried to make school an engaging place to be while having as much fun as possible along the way. Even when life's fortunes kicked me in the guts and brought me to my knees with cancer, I got back up when I was knocked down with the help of my faith, family, friends, my students, and staff. I will be able to look my two beautiful grandchildren in the eye one day and say, "Grandpa never gave in and never gave up." I can look in the mirror and know that I played the game the right way, leaving it all on the field, and have zero regrets.

Although I will dearly miss squaring up to the challenges facing us in the business of education today, what I will really miss are the little things. The relationships and stories (believe me, I've got a few) generated by working with my students, athletes, and their parents over the years, as well as the many friendships I have developed with my colleagues. What I will miss most of all is being a part of watching and impacting young people as they grow from being wide-eyed seventh graders into caring and responsible young adults. Having been a part of that in so many lives has been so rewarding for me. It's where I have felt most comfortable and free. It's where I am at ease and at peace. I don't know what could ever replace the feeling of being completely at home with young people while at work. To all my students, athletes and colleagues I have had the pleasure of working with and learning from over the years, it's you who I will think of when I reflect on the past forty years. It's you who have filled my heart and soul with so many laughs and so much love. I just want you to know that I love you all.

I was once asked by a teammate early in my playing days, if I didn't make it to the big leagues, would I consider my baseball playing days "all for naught"? I didn't hesitate as I said, "No way, it's about the journey and those who were a part of it along the way!" In the same way, the journey and relationships I have experienced in my education career have been a "Big League" experience! I look forward to teaching the lessons I have learned to my grandchildren and using those same lessons in the next phase of my life's journey and the many opportunities that will present as I continue to serve others.

My focus will be on family and wellness. I plan to continue advocating for After School Programming and Education at the state and national levels, my scouting work with the Atlanta Braves, tending our family farm, as well as serving others in Cedar Falls helping keep this area the best place to raise and educate a family in the State of Iowa. I look forward to my next adventure. I'm not sure which direction God will lead me, but I trust His plan and am excited to see what the next chapter has in store for me.

I will leave you with a thought from one of my favorite authors by the name of Jon Gordon. When writing one of his recent books, *The Carpenter,* he talked about being filled with the fear that he would disappoint the people who had enjoyed reading his previous books—fear that people would say his best writing was behind him, fears that he would write a piece of junk. At that moment, he realized the antidote to fear is love. So instead of the fear of failing, he decided to focus on his love of writing, his love for the reader, and his desire to make a difference. From that moment on the book flowed. He wrote it in two and a half weeks and discovered that if you focus on love, you will cast out fear.

I want to encourage each of you to do the same as you build your life, work, business, school, project, or team with love instead of fear. Remind yourself that if you aren't building it with love it won't become all that it can be. Only through love will you create something special, magnificent, and compelling. Only through love will you build a masterpiece.

As Jon shares, if you are trying to build a business, focus on the love you have of building it rather than the fear of losing it.

If you work at a school, focus on loving your students instead of fearing all the new testing standards and mandates. If you are a young athlete, dancer, musician or artist, focus on your love of playing and performing instead of your fear of failing. Worrying about the outcome and what people think will steal your joy and sabotage your success, but loving and appreciating the moment will energize you and enhance your performance. Love all of it!

Most of all, as Jon Gordon writes, "When you build with love, know that you will face many challenges and negative influences that can shift your focus back to fear if you let it. When this happens decide to **love all of it**. When you love all of it you will fear none of it."

Love the struggle because it makes you appreciate your accomplishments.
Love challenges because they make you stronger.
Love competition because it makes you better.
Love negative people because they make you more positive.
Love those who have hurt you because they teach you forgiveness.
Love fear because it makes you courageous.

The secret to life and the greatest success strategy of all is to love all of it and fear none of it! Thanks to all for taking this journey with me. I am, and have been, truly blessed.

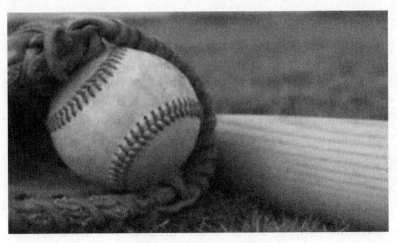

Hanging up My Cleats

An Encouraging Attitude

"All for naught?"
"No way!
It's about the journey and those who were a part of it
along the way!"

A Spiritual Insight

"Whatever you do, work at it with all your heart,
as working for the Lord, not for human masters."
(Colossians 3:23)

A Step to Consider

"The secret to life and the greatest success strategy of all is to love all of it and fear none of it!" – Jon Gordon

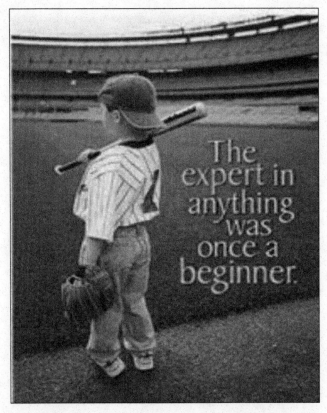

The Expert in Anything Was Once a Beginner

Reflection 41

New Beginnings

August 16, 2016

As I thought through my first reflection since retiring, I couldn't help but think back on all the times I was a beginner at whatever task was at hand. Experience is a great teacher, but we all have to begin somewhere. Young people looking to get into education often asked me the question, "Who will hire me if I don't have experience, and how am I supposed to get experience if they won't hire me?" Good question, but it comes down to focusing all your energy on building toward your goal, whatever that goal may be for you, one small step at a time.

As I recalled being a beginner as a student, athlete, parent, teacher, coach, an administrator, and yes, as a cancer survivor, it reminded me, "The expert in anything was once a beginner!" Experiencing all those journeys certainly made me no expert, but it did allow me the option of sharing what I've learned along the way as part of my new beginning in retirement.

> **"How lucky I am to have something that
> makes saying goodbye so hard..." — Pooh**

Change, new beginnings, and saying goodbye all wrapped up into one for me this past year. I'll begin by providing an update on my health situation. I've had several bumps in the road the past few months with lab readings and a cyst that appeared on one of my kidneys. So far, all seems stable and my doctors are monitoring both, so I feel comfortable that all is in good hands.

As for retirement, "How lucky I am to have something that makes saying goodbye so hard!" (Pooh). For the first time in forty years, I haven't been a part of the opening of a school year. Yes, I miss the students and staff who have been a part of this time of the year. Always knew I would. However, I've had the opportunity to fill that void by spending time with both of my beautiful granddaughters, Grace and Lucy. Brings back memories of my own three kids when they were that age.

**I've discovered that the secret of change is to focus
all of your energy
on building the new, not on fighting the old.**

For me, 2016 is the beginning of anything I choose! I am choosing to stay within the community of Cedar Falls, a place that I have come to know and love for many, many years. I plan to stay involved with scouting, educational consulting, and volunteering my time and services here in the community, and of course, spending more quality time with my family who I dearly love. To me, a perfect way to spend my retirement is to share what I've been fortunate enough to learn over the years by giving back without having the responsibilities I had when working. Retirement also allows me more time to read and reflect which has also been important to me over the years.

I just finished a profoundly moving memoir by a young neurosurgeon faced with a terminal cancer diagnosis. In his writing, he attempts to answer the question, "What makes a life worth living?" It's titled, *When Breath Becomes Air*, written by Paul Kalanithi.

At the age of thirty-six and on the verge of completing a decade's worth of training as a neurosurgeon, Paul was diagnosed with stage IV lung cancer. One day he was a doctor making a living treating the dying, and the next he was a patient struggling to live. Just like that, the future he and his wife had imagined evaporated. *When Breath Becomes Air* shares Kalanithi's transformation from being a naïve medical student to being possessed by the questions of what makes a virtuous and meaningful life.

What makes life worth living in the face of death?
What do you do when the future is no longer a ladder
toward your goals in life
as it flattens out into a perpetual present?

Many of the questions he asks in his book were the same questions I asked myself when faced with my cancer diagnosis. Interestingly, his insights also provided some good thoughts about how to make life meaningful, not only with the adjustments that are made as a cancer patient, but also with the adjustments we make when we pursue a new beginning such as in retirement.

Paul Kalanithi died in March 2015, while working on this book. His words will live on as a guide and a gift to us all. In his book, Paul quoted seven words from Samuel Beckett that he began repeating in his head once diagnosed with terminal cancer: "I can't go on. I will go on."

I've often felt the same, and it's comforting to know others also summon the drive to go on despite all odds seemingly going against us. *When Breath Becomes Air* is an unforgettable, life-affirming reflection on the challenge of facing mortality and on the relationship between doctor and patient, from a gifted writer who became both.

To close, I'm excited about my new beginning in my life. I'm hopeful my experiences will assist in making me an "expert" while helping make it meaningful for others on their life's journey.

An Encouraging Attitude

I've discovered that the secret of change
is to focus all of your energy on building the new,
not on fighting the old.

A Spiritual Insight

"But you, man of God, flee from all this,
and pursue righteousness, godliness, faith, love, endurance
and gentleness.
Fight the good fight of the faith.
Take hold of the eternal life to which you were called
when you made your good confession in the presence of
many witnesses."
(Apostle Paul to his disciple in 1 Timothy 6:11-12)

A Step to Consider

As you travel the new beginnings in each of your lives, remember, the expert in anything was once a beginner.

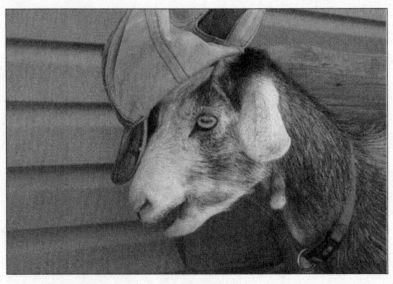

Scapegoating

Reflection 42

No Scapegoating!

October 18, 2016

S ome tests performed as part of my routine fall checkups indicated I needed to have a biopsy performed to see if the **Visiting Team** had returned for some extra inning competition. My mind again began wandering; wondering and projecting all kinds of thoughts about what the future may hold. I needed to remind myself that any thoughts about "future" things were actually thoughts about "secret" things, and these secret things belonged to the Lord.

My experiences over the past seven years have shown me that when I tried to grasp and understand the future, it was a futile act. Instead of worrying about the future, I needed to relax and enjoy my journey by opening up to and depending on God to guide me one step forward at a time. As our circumstances can often consume us, we need to discipline ourselves to live in the present moment so that we don't stagger under the load and stumble into home plate as we round the bases. Many times we turn to "scapegoating" and blaming others for our circumstances, which only serves as a distraction in resolving the real issues we may be facing.

We can always walk confidently through our toughest times knowing we are not alone! God and my **Home Team** have always been there for me, providing the love and support I've needed to make it through each day. As I watched the 2016 World Series, I couldn't help but draw some analogies between the success the Cubs had and the thoughts shared in this reflection.

I've always assumed that we feared the unknown. It's just one of those clichés that you hear so often that you just figure is true. Then last month, my mind opened to a very different possibility. After reading some thoughts from Steve Gilbert (*Win Your Day*), I concluded it's not the unknown that scares us. It is what we project into the unknown that causes our anxiety. That is because if something were truly unknown, we wouldn't know about it, so there wouldn't be any fear of it.

The more I thought about it, the more sense it made to me. I'm not so worried anymore about the unknown when it comes to my future. I'm worried about what my mind projects into the blank space that is the unknown. It may seem like semantics, but at least for me it had a big impact. It helped me to realize that it's my thoughts about things that scare, worry, and upset me rather than the things themselves.

For example, just take a look at a time in your life when you thought you were worried about the unknown— (for me that's easy, it's when I was diagnosed with cancer in 2009). See if what you were really worried about is what you projected might happen rather than simply not knowing what would. Once diagnosed, my mind began racing about many things and anxieties began sprouting up like mushrooms about what might happen, not what would happen. I shared many of those thoughts in my early reflections. My thoughts were often dominated by dealing with the pain, fear, and worry that accompany a serious medical diagnosis such as cancer.

I've discovered that the best defense against worry, fear or things that upset us is to stay in communication with God. By turning our thoughts to God when faced with these concerns, we can think more positively. By taking the time to think things through, then listening and discussing them with God instead of us being the "god" of our own thoughts and fantasies, we can experience much more satisfaction.

Quite often, the more hassled our lives become, the more we need time alone communing with God. He doesn't want us tied up in anxious knots, but rather to find peace in leaning on Him and remembering that He is our strength in those difficult times. This is not always easy because the world is often rigged to pull our attention away from Him. The noise and stimulations around us often make it hard to find Him in the midst of our difficult moments.

I've found another distraction during difficult times can be our own egos which so often want to project our pain and suffering onto another person or group. The term that applies here is "scapegoating." I can certainly relate to this having been both a scapegoat and having scapegoated others during my time as a teacher, coach, and principal. As I watch this year's baseball divisional playoffs, the Cubs come to mind.

Many diehard Chicago Cubs' fans have an unusual explanation for why their team hasn't been to a World Series in seven decades: a Billy goat. The superstition dates back to October 6, 1945, when a local bar owner supposedly placed a hex on the club for booting his foul-smelling pet goat out of Wrigley Field. The Cubs have struggled ever since, and have even earned the nickname the "lovable losers" for their perennial failure to win the World Series.

Think of the pain and suffering these die-hard fans have experienced over the years, which has at times been "scapegoated" to this curse. Recent Cubs management has showed us how to "hold the pain" and let it transform the team, rather than pass it on to the others around them by making good player personnel decisions and providing sound leadership. The results are speaking for themselves!

Spiritually and emotionally speaking, we can take a lesson from this. Don't be distracted from your situation by projecting pain and suffering onto another person or group. This can be difficult, believe me, as we face the future with a cancer or difficult medical diagnosis. There are no "bad goats to expel." I pray that I may be wise enough to identify my own problems, take them to God in prayer, and not be looking for the goats in others as I lean on Him for guidance while enjoying and relaxing in His presence during my difficult times.

When we have difficult moments which can cause pain and suffering in our lives, we need to take the time to bring them to God and ask for His guidance. Don't beat yourself up wondering "why me" or by projecting the pain and suffering onto others. Each day is a new day, it's a blank canvas, take them one at a time. Build off the lessons of yesterday, (just like the Cubs) without taking the frustration and upset into today.

An Encouraging Attitude

I've discovered that the best defense against worry, fear or
things that upset us
is to stay in communication with God.

A Spiritual Insight

"For God is not a God of disorder but of peace."
(1 Corinthians 14:33)

A Step to Consider

When you have difficult moments that cause pain and
suffering,
take the time to bring them to God and ask for His guidance.
Don't beat yourself up wondering "why me"
or by projecting the pain and suffering onto others.

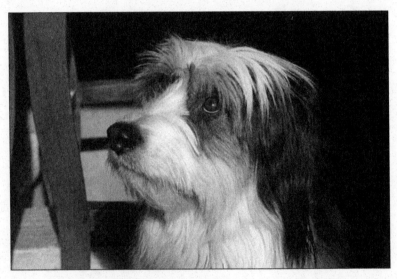

"Listening is an attitude of the heart." - L. J. Isham

Reflection 43

Listening Moment

December 9, 2016

My journey has taught me to focus on learning to listen to God, especially while we are listening to other people as they share their needs and concerns with us. By also listening to God during those times, He can think, live, and love through us as we respond to others. We need to use our time and energy to listen to and pray for others in their time of need as God offers His shielding presence whenever we are feeling fearful, experiencing threatening thoughts, and in need of a safe place sheltering us from those thoughts fears.

Jon Gordon said, "I've learned to talk to myself instead of listen to myself."

This may be one of the best pieces of advice I've ever received. If I "listen" to myself, I hear all the reasons why I should give up. I hear that I'm too tired, too old, and too weak to make it. But if I "talk" to myself, I can give myself the encouragement and words I need to hear to keep living out my journey here on earth in a positive way each and every day. Think about the power in this simple act of talking to yourself instead of listening to yourself.

When I wake up in the morning, do I immediately listen to my body telling me that I'm too tired to get out of bed and an extra 30 minutes of sleep is needed? Or do I instead talk to myself about the positive possibilities that the day will hold?

When a setback occurs like I have a poor performance, I lose a game, or I have a worrisome medical diagnosis, do I listen to the doubt and negative thoughts that can creep into my head? Or do I talk to myself about how much better things are going to be if I place my trust in God and approach each circumstance with a positive outlook and mindset?

I pray that throughout my day today and every day, I will be aware of whether I am listening to myself or talking to myself. It is a key difference between allowing circumstances to dictate our feelings or living our lives the way we want.

**"Listening is an attitude of the heart,
a genuine desire to be with another that both attracts and
heals." — L. J. Isham**

I have had several medical evaluations in Iowa City this past week. Results are mostly favorable at this point, which I am very thankful for. I have a follow up procedure scheduled in early January to deal with some polyps found this past fall, and hope to get that behind me soon. On a positive note, one of my doctors shared a new technology with regard to biopsies. It's called MRI-Fusion. It eliminates the need for **needles**! I'm certainly all for that!

Several thoughts ran through my mind as I sat and visited with an elderly gentleman in Iowa City this past week at one of my follow up appointments. He had so much to share about his life journey. It appeared what he really wanted was someone to just listen, so listen I did. He shared how he had been diagnosed with colon cancer a number of years ago, won the battle with treatments, and is now facing prostate cancer. He lost his wife along the way, his loving partner in life, which has made his journey more difficult and lonely, but he vowed to move on and remain positive about his situation.

Somehow the conversation drifted to the Cubs and their World Series victory this past year and he truly bubbled with joy as he has been a lifelong Cubs fan! He shared he much prefers listening to baseball on the radio as that is how he grew up, and it allows him to use his imagination in visualizing the game rather than be distracted by all the images on the T.V. I can relate as I also enjoy listening to games on the radio as I travel. It was a genuine "listening moment," which was good for both of us!

My first thought after our conversation was that problems are a part of life. Pretty obvious, I know. What I reflected on is that problem solving has been a daily part of my life as a teacher, coach, school principal, and cancer survivor. I literally go into "problem solving mode" immediately when faced with a challenge. I guess that is not all bad if kept in proper perspective. It can often weigh me down, though, as I have sometimes taken on responsibilities that are not my own. When engaged in problem solving, I need to remind myself to keep looking to God for strength and guidance, as He will provide the armor needed to help me stand my ground and handle the difficulties that come my way.

Another thought that entered my mind was that "listening" rather than "fixing" could be a great way to deal with problems we face. Listening can be a lost art in this era of social media where we are so used to sharing our thoughts and opinions. I thought this morning about how often I am not really listening to what a person is telling me, but rather just waiting for them to stop talking so I can share what I have to say. My work driving at Western Home Communities has really helped me to learn to listen to folks. They truly appreciate a listening ear and I have really learned a lot by just listening.

I used to worry that there would be times when I wouldn't have answers for people who sought my assistance. After spending time with the residents, I have come to realize that what people want more than anything is to be heard. Most times they don't need you to tell them what to do; they want your help in discovering it for themselves and that comes from asking questions and then really listening to what they have to say.

When taking these folks to medical appointments, they don't feel you need to heal them. They don't expect you to remove their pain or have some great words of wisdom, but rather to hold their hand, listen, and be present. That is comforting to both them and to me.

After reading Steve Gilbert's, *Win Your Day,* I am working hard at learning to listen with my heart, and trying to make wise choices while making it my goal to be positive, helpful, and hopeful to those around me. Sometimes, I just literally have to tell myself, "Just put the glove down and listen!"

Having spent a lot of time in Iowa City and talking there to many who are struggling with health issues, I've found there is something incredibly powerful about a person who cannot be defeated. Everyone loses at some point in their lives, but whether or not that loss defeats you is under your control. If I'm feeling discouraged, frustrated or having other negative feelings, I need to let those emotions remind me that joy and being positive are choices, and I can choose to be positive and hopeful moment by moment.

How you react to the loss of a job, a loss in competition, the way someone has treated you or even the loss of the health and physical wellbeing you have always enjoyed is up to you! Don't put your head down and give up, and don't choose to play the victim recounting to your friends over and over how you were wronged.

As we all face our individual challenges, we need to remember each day to continue to choose not to be defeated. Allow some reflective time in acknowledging a loss, allow yourself to feel the disappointment of that loss, but take a hard look at the situation for what you can learn from it to be better in the future. Bottom line, don't be defeated and don't play the victim! As Steve points out, "Reclaim your power to live life from the inside out!" Keep moving forward with your head up and continue to develop your ability to lose yet never be defeated.

An Encouraging Attitude

If I'm feeling discouraged, frustrated or other negative feelings,
I need to let those emotions remind me that joy and
being positive are choices,
and I can choose to be positive and hopeful moment
by moment.

A Spiritual Insight

"Therefore put on the full armor of God,
so that when the day of evil comes,
you may be able to stand your ground,
and after you have done everything, to stand."
(Secrets to victory from Ephesians 6:13)

A Step to Consider

Choose not to be defeated.
Allow some reflective time in acknowledging a loss,
allow yourself to feel the disappointment of that loss,
but take a hard look at the situation for what you
can learn from it
to be better in the future.
Bottom line, don't be defeated and don't play the victim!

249

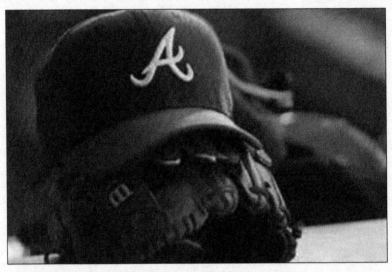

Sometimes I have to tell myself, "just put the glove down and listen!"

Closing Reflection

February 27, 2017

A s I close my personal reflections, please remember God designed us to live close to Him so that by trusting in Him we can feel peaceful and complete. Sometimes, we tend to forget this as we deal with life's challenges on our own instead of staying in touch with Him.

I feel that the very things that have often troubled me most, my personal weaknesses and wounds, can be used in helping others. By letting these humble, hurting parts of me be exposed, I'm hopeful they can help others by letting God's light and guidance enter their lives through my experiences.

By receiving God's healing, loving, and guiding presence during those times of weakness and wounding in our lives, and in turn revealing them to others, we can help minister and comfort those who may be experiencing the same struggles. God's strength comes into its own in our weaknesses. The two fit together perfectly.

That takes me to a note I received late this past fall from a person who had my journal forwarded to her by a mutual friend as she was battling cancer.

Her note in part read:

> "Your reflections gave me strength when I was dying. I just wanted to thank you for giving me

hope and strength. As I was fighting cancer over the past year, I read your reflections while I was in the hospital. Your words kept my spirits high when I needed it most. And believe it or not, the 25% estimated chance of survival they gave me 12 months ago became 99.9% this morning when my doctors officially concluded that my cancer is in complete remission. I'm just so grateful I get to use some of the thoughts you shared in my second chance at life."

Above all else, her note reminded me that too many of us wait too long to live our best lives. We keep putting every-thing off until tomorrow. Then, before we know it, we find ourselves asking, "How did it get so late so soon?" We need to take time to love, laugh, cry, learn, and forgive. Life is often shorter than it seems.

A final thought written by Chuck Swindoll titled, *Friendly People, Thoughtful People,* lovingly describes the special people who have sur-rounded me in my life, making up my precious **Home Team.**

"If I have learned anything during my journey on Planet Earth, it is that people need one another.

The presence of other people is essential —caring people, helpful people, interesting people, friendly people, and thoughtful people. These folks take the grind out of life.

About the time we are tempted to think we can handle things all alone —boom! We run into some obstacle and need assistance. We dis-cover all over again that we are not nearly as self-sufficient as we thought.

In spite of our high-tech world and efficient procedures, people remain the essential ingredient of life. When we forget that, a strange thing happens: We start treating people like inconveniences instead of assets."

May each of your lives be filled with personal reflection and reaching out to others by sharing His unfailing love for each of us.

Preparing for the "Post-Season"

One of my goals as a coach was to always review with my players a fundamentals checklist as the regular season came to a close each year. The checklist was intended to highlight a series of specific fundamentals we had learned from instruction and experiences during the regular season. It provided a takeaway for my players to carry with them into tournament play, with a goal of helping us to be successful as we played into the post season. Just as this checklist was helpful to my teams, I wanted to provide readers with a post-season checklist as you, a family member or friend travel their life's journey facing the challenges life may present. The following checklist of encouraging attitudes, spiritual insights, and steps to consider have helped provide me with some basic "fundamentals" which I have found to be useful throughout my cancer experience and as I enter my post-season journey as a cancer survivor. May they do the same for you and those you love.

"Encouraging Attitudes" Fundamental Check List

✓ Have a game plan for each day, beginning each with a clean slate.

✓ When faced with a difficult situation like cancer, or for that matter any tough situation, it is so important to reach out to others for help and support.

✓ Live in the present, taking one day at a time while revolving any thoughts encountered around hope!

✓ Make a guarantee to yourself that nowhere in your story will it ever read, "I gave up!"

✓ Keep your sense of humor! Laughter is a great healer.

✓ No matter what anyone says, just show up and do the work!

✓ Refuse to grow discouraged by communing with God who helps provide the nutrients to grow the strength and courage to make it through!

✓ Always turn a negative into a positive leaving in its place something gained not lost!

✓ Failure equips us to value learning and to relish challenge and effort while using those errors as routes to mastery.

✓ **Nothing can stop the man with the right mental attitude from achieving his goal.**

✓ God is always there, "never blinking" at the challenges we are presented and will help carry us through difficult times.

✓ Take a neutral attitude towards the things you cannot control.

✓ God's purpose for us is not to grant our every wish, making my life easy and pain free, but rather to allow us to learn to trust Him in all circumstances.

✓ Don't take the easy way out! Stay in control, using courage and conviction to face any suffering and challenges you may face.

✓ Even though cancer may invade your body, never let it invade your soul!

✓ Worry is defined as a matter of thinking about things at the wrong time.

✓ My encouragement to any cancer patient or anyone struggling with emotional pain, is remember it is important not to ignore the emotional side of suffering. The advice, "Just suck it up" doesn't work.

✓ Where the heart is willing, it will find a thousand ways, but where it is unwilling it will find a thousand excuses.

✓ No matter how "bumpy the ride" and even though we may not fully understand His plan, God is preparing us for a far better place than this.

✓ When everything seems like it's falling apart, that's when God is putting things together just the way He wants it!

✓ Never lose your determination, it is just too important, and it's truly what drives us.

✓ "You'll get through this. It won't be painless. It won't be quick. But God will use this mess for good. Don't be foolish or naïve. But don't despair either. With God's help, you'll get through this." - *Art of Living* by Max Lucado

✓ We all have more work to do according to God's plan!

✓ "Remember, life gives us warnings for a reason. Learn from this. Do things differently." - Jon Gordon from his book, *"The Carpenter."*

✓ "To be successful, you have to fix your eyes and focus on the ball, blocking out all those things that may be whirling around in your mind competing for your focus and attention." - Coach John Paulsen

✓ Setbacks can help plant the seeds for new dreams in each of our lives and provide great life lessons for each of us.

✓ "We can't let yesterday take up too much of today." – Will Rogers

✓ Don't allow the temptation of quick shortcuts to fool you as you move forward toward your personal wellness goals

✓ God's plan for each of us may not always save us from something, but He may be saving us for something!

✓ Life is all about the journey and those who were a part of it along the way!

✓ I've discovered that the secret of change is to focus all of your energy on building the new, not on fighting the old.

✓ I've also discovered that the best defense against worry, fear or things that upset us is to stay in communication with God.

"Spiritual Insights" Fundamental Check List

✓ "Therefore do not worry about tomorrow, for tomorrow will worry about itself.
Each day has enough trouble of its own." (Jesus teaching in Matthew 6:34) (Jesus in John 10:10)

✓ "Be joyful in hope, patient in affliction, faithful in prayer." (Paul's instructions for dealing with life's difficulties Romans 12:12)

✓ "[The Lord] gives strength to the weary and increases the power of the weak." (Isaiah 40:29)

✓ "Do you not know that in a race all the runners run, but only one gets the prize?
Run in such a way as to get the prize."(Paul's advice in 1 Corinthians 9:24)

✓ "For I know the plans I have for you," declares the LORD, "plans to prosper you and not to harm you, plans to give you hope and a future."(Jeremiah 29:11)

✓ "The thief comes only in order to steal and kill and destroy. I came that they may have *and* enjoy life, and have it in abundance [to the full, till it overflows]." (Jesus in John 10:10)

✓ "Love never fails. And now these three remain: faith, hope and love.
But the greatest of these is love." (Promise from God in 1 Corinthians 13:8, 13)

✓ "Whoever dwells in the shelter of the Most High will rest in the shadow of the Almighty. I will say of the LORD, He is my refuge and my fortress, my God, in whom I trust." (David as he teaches us to deal with life's issues in Psalm 91:1-2)

✓ "Suffering produces perseverance." (Romans 5:3)

✓ "Therefore, if anyone is in Christ, the new creation has come: The old has gone, the new is here!" (2 Corinthians 5:17)

✓ "God is our refuge and strength, an ever-present help in trouble." (Psalm 46:1)

✓ "Base your happiness on your hope in Christ. When trials come endure them patiently, steadfastly maintain the habit of prayer."[9] (Romans 12:12)

✓ "My dear brothers and sisters, take note of this: Everyone should be quick to listen, slow to speak and slow to become angry, because human anger does not produce the righteousness that God desires." (James the brother of Jesus in James 1:19-20)

✓ "For we know that if the earthly tent we live in is destroyed, we have a building from God, an eternal house in heaven, not built by human hands."(2 Corinthians 5:1)

✓ "So we fix our eyes not on what is seen, but on what is unseen, since what is seen is temporary, but what is unseen is eternal." (2 Corinthians 4:18)

---

[9]

✓ "But in your hearts revere Christ as Lord. Always be prepared to give an answer to everyone who asks you to give the reason for the hope that you have. But do this with gentleness and respect." (1 Peter 3:15)

✓ "I have told you these things, so that in me you may have peace. In this world you will have trouble. But take heart! I have overcome the world." (Jesus in John 16:33)

✓ "Do everything without grumbling or arguing, so that you may become blameless and pure, children of God without fault in a warped and crooked generation. Then you will shine among them like stars in the sky." (Apostle Paul while in a Roman prison - Philippians 2:14-15)

✓ "Consider it pure joy my brothers and sisters, whenever you face trials of many kinds, because you know that the testing of your faith produces perseverance."(-James 1:2-3)

✓ "But thanks be to God! He gives us the victory through our Lord Jesus Christ. Therefore, my dear brothers and sisters, stand firm. Let nothing move you." (1 Corinthians 15:57-58)

✓ "Forget the former things; do not dwell on the past." (God to His people in Isaiah 43:18)]

✓ "But thanks be to God! He gives us the victory through our Lord Jesus Christ. Therefore, my dear brothers and sisters, stand firm. Let nothing move you." (1 Corinthians 15:57-58)

✓ "Whatever you do, work at it with all your heart, as working for the Lord, not for human masters." (Colossians 3:23)

✓ "For God is not a God of disorder but of peace." (1 Corinthians 14:33)

✓ "Therefore put on the full armor of God, so that when the day of evil comes, you may be able to stand your ground, and after you have done everything, to stand." (Secrets to victory from Ephesians 6:13)

"Steps to Consider" Fundamental Check List

✓ Gather a Support Team around you while you work to develop your game plan.

✓ Don't let the "**Visiting Team**" dictate your emotions. Be positive and proactive, not negative and reactive as you move onward.

✓ Reading will bring much encouragement and comfort on your journey. Read an encouraging book and be inspired!

✓ Use education and its relevance in your daily life to think outside the box and tackle problems by using **all** the resources at your disposal.

✓ Don't wait for a major life event to happen to you, make a plan for your life and set it out in small attainable goals — starting today.

✓ Take care of your body. Keep it well fed and watered.

✓ Stay focused and patient as you go through the process, no matter what the challenge!

✓ Read God's word and find the support you need for the journey from God. His love can free you from fear, anger, anxieties, and the troubles you face in this life.

✓ Be open about your struggles. Seek out friends as a means of support to provide hope and comfort.

✓ Spend some personal quiet time with God in the Scriptures each day and experience God's unfailing love.

✓ The Lord and His angels are always there, but so are friends and family. Be sure to access them.

✓ Don't waste energy on what cannot be changed.

✓ Continue to play the game hard no matter what cards you are dealt.

✓ Anger doesn't change circumstances

- ✓ Share those thoughts and feelings with God, He always listens.
- ✓ "Minor league thinking" results in major league benefits.
- ✓ Take charge of your thoughts each day. Remember, you will find God when you seek Him above all else.
- ✓ Remember to hang on just a little while longer. Focus only on the task that is right in front of you.
- ✓ Be prepared. Luck is truly where preparation meets opportunity.
- ✓ You can have an impact on others who may be facing similar trials and afflictions by modeling a positive and determined attitude in your own battle.
- ✓ As you live out your life embracing the gifts you have been given and rising up to meet the challenges you are faced with, remember, "Tough times don't last, but tough people do... if we keep hoping!"
- ✓ Place your troubles in God's hands and allow Him to be in control.
- ✓ Instead of complaining when hardships come your way, lean on those **Home Team** members and show your gratitude for their help.
- ✓ If you get knocked down, pick yourself up. If someone else gets knocked down, help pick him or her up.
- ✓ Focus away from the problem altogether and place it back on Jesus to be refreshed in His daily presence.
- ✓ Take every opportunity to continue to experience the simple joys that life brings. Joys such as hugging your spouse, children, and grandchildren.
- ✓ "The secret to life and the greatest success strategy of all is to love all of it and fear none of it!" – Jon Gordon
- ✓ As you travel the new beginnings in each of your lives, remember, the expert in anything was once a beginner.
- ✓ When you have difficult moments that cause pain and suffering, take the time to bring them to God and

ask for His guidance. Don't beat yourself up wondering "why me."

✓ Allow some reflective time in acknowledging a loss, allow yourself to feel the disappointment of that loss, but take a hard look at the situation for what you can learn from it to be better in the future. Bottom line, don't be defeated and don't play the victim!

Acknowledgments

S haring my thoughts while traveling my cancer journey has been a "from the heart" experience, allowing me to process and reflect on the many emotions and fears that have invaded my mind since this adventure began back in 2009. As you can tell from reading those thoughts, not all of them have been positive, but with the help of my **Home Team** I have strived to make them productive.

Many people have been a special part of my **Home Team** including family, friends, colleagues, my students, and staff as well as the many authors whom I have had the privilege to read and relate with along the way. I give special thanks to them all for helping me remain upbeat and encouraging me to share the thoughts and reflections in this book. I also want to thank my Church family for their positive and encouraging support throughout the journey. A special thanks is extended to my editor, Dr. Larry Keefauver and his team at Xulon press for "coaching me" through this process. Being a "rookie" author, his suggestions have been extremely helpful in helping me craft my thoughts and share them with all of you. Dr. Larry and his team have been a blessing to me in this project.

It is my prayer that these reflections may help others find their way when dealing with the struggles each day can bring while always keeping God at their side along the way. Most importantly, I want to thank Jesus Christ who has taught me through this trial to,

"Be joyful in hope, patient in affliction, and faithful in prayer" (Romans 12:12).

About the Author

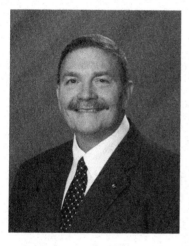

David Welter recently retired from the Cedar Falls Community School District in Cedar Falls, Iowa, after serving forty years in education, thirty-seven of which were spent in Cedar Falls. During that time, he taught social studies, has been involved with baseball at the high school, college, and professional levels, while also serving as a Jr. High principal for the past sixteen years.

Since retiring, Welter continues to scout for the Atlanta Braves, works as an education consultant, farms, and enjoys precious time with his children and granddaughters. Welter has been inducted into the Iowa High School Baseball Coaches Hall of Fame as well as being named Iowa's Middle Level Principal of the Year in 2013.

Image Bibliography - *Reflections from the Home Team; Go the Distance*

March 2, 2009; Personal photo
March 5, 2009; Pixabay royalty free image

March 13, 2009; Pixabay royalty free image
March 20, 2009; Permission granted by Hope Lodge
March 27, 2009; Pixabay royalty free image
April 3, 2009; Pixabay royalty free image
April 9, 2009; Pixabay royalty free image
April 17, 2009; Pixabay royalty free image
April 24, 2009; Pixabay royalty free image
May 1, 2009; Pixabay royalty free image
May 8, 2009; purchased Dreamstime_m_83351341 (1).jpg
June 3, 2009; Personal photo
August 9, 2009; Pixabay royalty free image
March 1, 2010; Pixabay royalty free image
March 27, 2010; Personal photo
May 20, 2010; Personal photo purchased – Head of Christ by Hook;
Matthew F Sheehan Co. SKU 200-1571-200-1571
August 21, 2010; Personal photo
November 14, 2010; Personal photo
February 13, 2011; Personal photo
February 23, 2011; Pixabay royalty free image
April 17, 2011; The Mick Mickey Mantle by Iconic Images Art Gallery David Pucciarelli Digital Download Royalty Free License #1342646
September 19, 2011; Pixabay royalty free image
December 10, 2011; Pixabay royalty free image
February 26, 2012; Personal photo
April 30, 2012; Pixabay royalty free image
July 26, 2012; Pixabay royalty free image
August 26, 2012; Pixabay royalty free image
November 4, 2012; Pixabay royalty free image
February 24, 2013; Royalty free image from http://z3news. com/w/wp - content/uploads/2015/04/corrie-ten-boom.jpg
June 1, 2013; purchased Dreamstime.com - robinson-
<href="https://www.dreamstime.com/stock-photography-trib- ute-to-jacke-image17963342#res17800914">Tribute to Jacke Robinson</a>

August 2, 2013; Royalty free Image from https://2.bp.blog-
  spot.com/-
N0ca9FU4RzI/WES7MzB-lVI/
  AAAAAAAAWw/23Spo_4U2pkb7iCHrUqAGm_
  gOjXMLNVqwCLcB/s1600/August+2,+2013.jpg
October 7, 2013; Personal photo
February 23, 2014; purchased Dreamstime.com - <a
href="https://www.dreamstime.com/royalty-free-
  stock-photos-curt-schilling-boston-red-sox-im-
  age17844278#res17800914">Curt Schilling Boston Red
  Sox Photo</a>
May 17, 2014; Royalty free image: Dreamstime.com - ID
  74577096 © Jerry Coli |
October 26, 2014;   Royalty free image from:
http://www2.ljworld.com/news/2014/oct/29/
  world-series-royals-game-7/
January 7, 2015; Royalty free image: http://dayandadream.
  com/wp-content/uploads/2014/07/stuart-scott-espys.jpg
May 16, 2015; purchased Dreamstime.com - <a href="https://
  www.dreamstime.com/editorial-image-greg-maddux-at-
  lanta-braves-former-pitcher-image-taken-color-slide-im-
  age57843905#res17800914">Greg Maddux Atlanta
  Braves</a>
October 10, 2015; Pixabay royalty free image
January 2, 2016; Royalty free image: https://3.bpblogspot.
  com/-RI4W_c4IM/V7pt3nifvl/AAAAAAAAUo/zInZ-
  FUyhZVQXMEdF_P-XEkND9eRheOoCWCLcB/s1600/
  UNTITLED.png
April 2, 2016; Pixabay royalty free image
April 16, 2016; Personal photo and Pixabay royalty
  free image
August 16, 2016; Personal poster - mpm school supplies –
  purchase order # A229473563, Product # 17425
October 18, 2016; Pixabay royalty free image
December 9, 2016; Pixabay royalty free image and per-
  sonal photo

February 27, 2017; Pixabay royalty free image
An Eagle Named Freedom
My True Story of a Remarkable Friendship
By Jeff Guidry

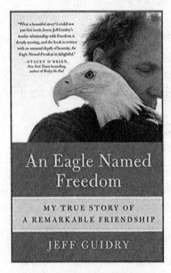

https://www.harpercollins.com/9780062015501/
an-eagle-named-freedom#

CPSIA information can be obtained
at www.ICGtesting.com
Printed in the USA
BVOW03s2156110717
489116BV00001B/52/P